WOMEN'S STRENGTH TRAINING ANATOMY

Library of Congress Cataloging-in-Publication Data

Delavier, Frédéric.
 [Exercises pour une belle ligne. English]
 Women's strength training anatomy / Frédéric Delavier.
    p. cm.
Rev. ed. of: Exercises pour une belle ligne. Paris : Editions Vigot,
2002.
Companion book to Strength training anatomy.
 ISBN 0-7360-4813-8 (soft cover)
 1. Muscles--Anatomy. 2. Women--Anatomy. 3. Weight training for
women. 4. Muscle strength. I. Delavier, Frédéric. Strength training
anatomy. II. Title.
 QM151 .D4513 2003
 611'.73--dc21

                            2002151925

ISBN-10: 0-7360-4813-8
ISBN-13: 978-0-7360-4813-2

Copyright © 2003 by Éditions Vigot, 23 rue de l'École de Médecine, 75006 Paris, France

This book is a revised edition of *Exercises Pour Une Belle Ligne,* published in 2002 by Éditions Vigot.

Acquisitions Editor: Martin Barnard
Managing Editors: Leigh LaHood and Julie A. Marx
Translator: Robert H. Black R.M.T.
Cover Designer: Keith Blomberg
Illustrator: Frédéric Delavier

Human Kinetics books are available at special discounts for bulk purchase. Special editions or book excerpts can also be created to specification. For details, contact the Special Sales Manager at Human Kinetics.

Printed in France by Pollina, n° L41183   10

Human Kinetics
Web site: www.HumanKinetics.com

United States: Human Kinetics
P.O. Box 5076
Champaign, IL 61825-5076
800-747-4457
e-mail: humank@hkusa.com

Canada: Human Kinetics
475 Devonshire Road Unit 100
Windsor, ON N8Y 2L5
800-465-7301 (in Canada only)
e-mail: orders@hkcanada.com

Europe: Human Kinetics
107 Bradford Road
Stanningley
Leeds LS28 6AT, United Kingdom
+44 (0) 113 255 5665
e-mail: hk@hkeurope.com

Australia: Human Kinetics
57A Price Avenue
Lower Mitcham, South Australia 5062
08 8277 1555
e-mail: liaw@hkaustralia.com

New Zealand: Human Kinetics
Division of Sports Distributors NZ Ltd.
P.O. Box 300 226 Albany
North Shore City
Auckland
0064 9 448 1207
e-mail: info@humankinetics.co.nz

WOMEN'S STRENGTH TRAINING ANATOMY

Frédéric Delavier

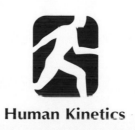

Human Kinetics

SOMMAIRE

KNOW YOUR BODY BETTER
TO TRAIN BETTER

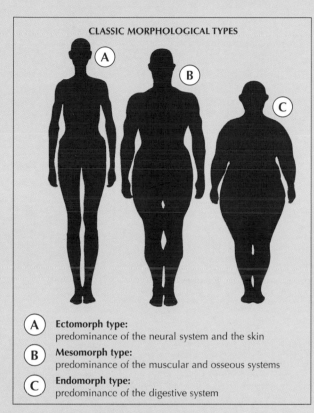

CLASSIC MORPHOLOGICAL TYPES

A **Ectomorph type:**
predominance of the neural system and the skin

B **Mesomorph type:**
predominance of the muscular and osseous systems

C **Endomorph type:**
predominance of the digestive system

PREDOMINANT BODY TYPES

To know your body better so that you train better, you must understand some basic concepts.

The embryo from which each of us is derived is the result of the fertilization of an ovum by a spermatozoa. Toward the end of the second week of this embryo's development three primitive layers are already outlined: the outer layer, called ectoderm; the middle layer, called mesoderm; and the deep layer, called endoderm. Each of these layers gives rise to very specific parts of the organism.

• The ectoderm forms both the epidermis, the sensory organs, the central nervous system, and the peripheral nerves.
• The mesoderm mainly forms the bones and muscles, the urogenital organs, the cardiovascular system, and the blood.
• The endoderm forms the intestinal mucosa and related glands.

The predominance of one of these three layers during growth provides the person with a well-defined body type.

PREDOMINANT ECTODERM DEVELOPMENT: ECTOMORPH TYPE

Ectomorphs appear fragile and delicate; they are lean and narrow in the shoulders. Although they are slender, their skeletons are prominent and the almost complete absence of fat reveals all the fibers of the muscle system even when it is not very developed.

Ectomorphs' thyroids are generally hyperactive, which accelerates their metabolisms so that they need to consume a lot of calories to maintain weight. Many ectomorphs who try to fill out can train daily because their bodies recuperate quickly, but they need a well balanced diet with foods rich in protein. To gain weight they must consume more calories than they expend, which does not happen automatically. Ectomorphs often lack muscle tone, and they commonly have vertebral pathologies (kyphosis, lordosis, scoliosis), the result of lack of strength in the erector muscles of the spine and the abdominal muscles. The weakness of the abdominals, moreover, is often responsible for ptosis of the lower part of the abdomen, which is no longer able to retain the viscera. Therefore, ectomorphs need to increase their muscle tone to correct postural defects.

ORGANS DERIVED FROM ECTODERM

◆ Epidermis, hair, nails, and cutaneous glands
◆ Mucosa of the oral, nasal, vaginal, and anal cavities
◆ Neural tissue
◆ Sensory organs
◆ Tooth enamel
◆ Lenses of the eyes
◆ Adrenal glands

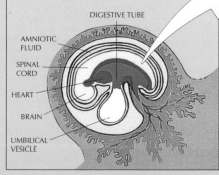

DIGESTIVE TUBE
AMNIOTIC FLUID
SPINAL CORD
HEART
BRAIN
UMBILICAL VESICLE

INTRODUCTION

PREDOMINANT MESODERM DEVELOPMENT: MESOMORPH TYPE

Mesomorphs tend to be muscular persons with large bones and thick joints. They have big clavicles and muscular shoulders, which give them a burly appearance. Their rib cages are well developed relative to their waistlines, in contrast to the endomorph's large waist. One of the striking features of the mesomorph is the well-developed musculature of the distal segments of their extremities; that is, they have powerful calves and forearms that can equal the thickness of the upper arms.

Because one of the effects of testosterone, the main hormone secreted by the testicles, is to increase muscle mass, naturally a large proportion of mesomorphs are men. On the other hand, testosterone is also secreted, although in lesser quantity, by the adrenal glands (the small glands capping the kidneys), so some women are also muscular mesomorph types because of the increased activity of these glands. Nevertheless, their development never matches that of male mesomorphs.

If the mesomorph type is more frequent in men, it is because natural selection, operating during millions of years of evolution, selected the most vigorous males: those capable of hunting, protecting the females and their offspring from external dangers, and maintaining dominance among their fellows for access to females. For this adaptation the male body tended toward expending energy (with powerful muscles and bones, well-developed heart and arteries) to respond to the intense activity men had to engage in to survive and reproduce. The lives of men have certainly changed a lot, but millions of years of evolution aren't erased overnight.

Mesomorphs often need to be active. If they are successful at most sports, however, their relatively significant muscle mass is somewhat of a handicap in endurance activities such as long-distance running. Only when they overeat do mesomorphs develop weight problems, whereas even moderate training allows them to maintain a toned athletic physique.

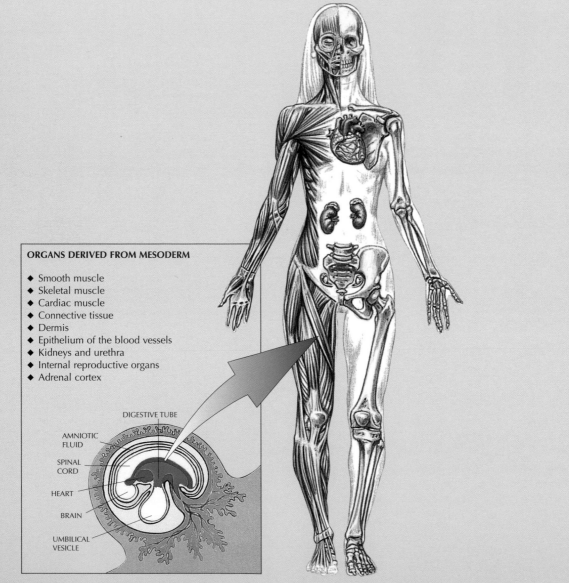

ORGANS DERIVED FROM MESODERM

- ◆ Smooth muscle
- ◆ Skeletal muscle
- ◆ Cardiac muscle
- ◆ Connective tissue
- ◆ Dermis
- ◆ Epithelium of the blood vessels
- ◆ Kidneys and urethra
- ◆ Internal reproductive organs
- ◆ Adrenal cortex

DIGESTIVE TUBE

AMNIOTIC FLUID

SPINAL CORD

HEART

BRAIN

UMBILICAL VESICLE

PREDOMINANT ENDODERM DEVELOPMENT: ENDOMORPH TYPE

Barring pathological obesity, endomorphs tend to be chubby. The development of their fat layer erases the muscle outline, which gives them a soft appearance. Osseous indicators are not evident, and the endomorphs' extremities are hamlike, coming to a point with relatively predominant thighs and upper arms above the calves and forearms. Although endomorphs' skeletons are not as fine as those of ectomorphs, they are also not as massive as those of mesomorphs.

The greater development of their digestive systems gives them a thick, sometimes potbellied, waist as if the metabolism of their entire bodies tends toward absorption. The endomorph type is more frequent in women, whose digestive systems are proportionately more developed and in whom fat is more abundant (under the effect of certain female hormones produced by the ovaries).

If women have more fat, it is because each woman's body is prepared to carry and feed a child from her own reserves, and consequently has to stockpile energy in the form of fat in case of eventual pregnancy.

Unlike ectomorphs, endomorphs have lazy thyroids: Their metabolism is slow and recovers more slowly than the other body types. On the other hand, they don't need to eat a lot, which is a significant advantage during scarcity; however, to lose weight for aesthetic reasons, they often must follow draconian diets that ultimately lead to nutritional deficiencies incompatible with good health.

Endomorphs rarely have back problems; their spines are swaddled by the significant volume of their torsos and have adapted to the masses they must support by losing part of their curves, which give them a columnar shape. On the other hand, endomorphs frequently have knee problems. In fact, the significant volume that they have acquired before the end of their growth—a period during which the bones maintain a certain suppleness—deforms their legs, which are often in an X (genu valgus), a condition that can create problems.

To keep in shape and to try to limit the amount of fat they carry, endomorphs need to combine regular training with a strict diet while taking care not to overtrain and avoiding nutritional deficiencies.

ORGANS DERIVED FROM ENDODERM

- Epithelium of the external auditory canal, tonsils, thyroid, parathyroid, thymus, larynx, tracheal artery, and lungs
- Digestive tract
- Bladder, urethra, and vagina
- Liver and pancreas

DIGESTIVE TUBE
AMNIOTIC FLUID
SPINAL CORD
HEART
BRAIN
UMBILICAL VESICLE

It must be said that pure ectomorph, mesomorph, or endomorph types do not exist; a person is most often a mixture of all three in various proportions, with one or two types predominating. The sprinter is often a mesomorph-ectomorph; the shot-putter a mesomorph-endomorph; the model with a svelte and slender profile more of an ectomorph, as is the long-distance runner.

The important point is to learn to recognize your individual predominance so that you can design an appropriate training program. One morphological type cannot be changed into another, but appropriate training can help people tone up by limiting the development of fat while firming up the predominant shape and then, secondarily, toning and building muscle.

FAT IN WOMEN

One of the main morphological differences between men and women is the greater amount of fat that women carry; this softens the outline of the muscles, more or less erases the osseous indicators, and rounds out the surfaces while creating characteristic folds and grooves.

Fat in normal women represents between 18% and 20% of body weight, whereas in men it represents only 10% to 15%. The reason for this difference is that women at some point in their lives may nourish a fetus and then a baby from their own reserves, so women have to stock energy in the form of fat in anticipation of future pregnancies (and must stock even more energy during the last two trimesters of pregnancy).

For various reasons, different fat distributions occur in women according to climate. In hot countries, the fat is localized on the buttocks (black Africans), on the hips (Mediterraneans), and around the navel (certain Asians). This distribution avoids covering the woman with a hot coat of fat that would be difficult to bear and inefficient for thermoregulation during hot periods. In cold countries, the distribution of fat is more uniform, which provides for better protection during rigorous winters. However the fat is distributed, its main function is for the survival of the species as it provides for survival of the woman and her offspring during times of scarcity.

It is important to note that all healthy people have fat reserves necessary for the proper functioning of their bodies. Obsession with obesity or the need to follow deviant aesthetic fashions should not lead to the complete elimination of fat. In fact, the almost complete disappearance of fat can lead to serious hormonal problems involving the cessation of the period (amenorrhea, which is a temporary absence of ovulation and therefore momentary sterility), as this means has been put in place during evolution to avoid bringing progeny into the world that the female could not nourish with her own organic reserves.

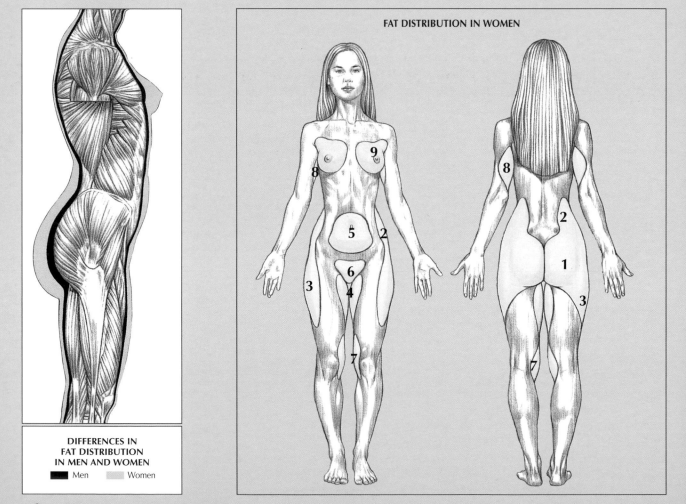

DIFFERENCES IN
FAT DISTRIBUTION
IN MEN AND WOMEN
■ Men ▢ Women

FAT DISTRIBUTION IN WOMEN

PRIMARY FAT DEPOSITS

Fat reserves accumulate in very specific areas on the body. Generally they avoid the flexion folds at the joints in order not to interfere with movement. Fat accumulations are often distributed the same in both sexes; the main difference is in the greater development on certain areas in women.

1. THE BUTTOCKS

The buttock region can be quite prominent in women; this is almost entirely due to fat that is contained by the gluteal fold. Besides its role as an energy reserve, this concentration protects the anal area and helps make the sitting position more comfortable by cushioning the direct contact between the bones (ischial tuberosities) and the ground or supporting surface.

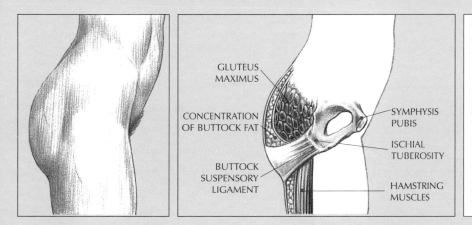

GLUTEUS MAXIMUS

CONCENTRATION OF BUTTOCK FAT

BUTTOCK SUSPENSORY LIGAMENT

SYMPHYSIS PUBIS

ISCHIAL TUBEROSITY

HAMSTRING MUSCLES

THE GLUTEAL FOLD

The gluteal fold is made up of tough, fibrous tracts that connect the deep surface of the skin in the gluteal area to the ischium. The main consequence of this fibrous attachment is to contain the fat in a sort of pocket, which prevents it from falling down against the back of the thigh while at the same time increasing the volume of the buttock. When certain people age, this fat empties and the bottom of the buttock withers, even going so far as to hang down. Only appropriate training of the buttock area will compensate for the disappearance of fat and the loss of tone through muscle development that maintains the buttocks from the inside.

2. LOW BACK

Second in importance, this concentration merges with the gluteal area so that the buttock increases in height until it seems to go up to the waist.

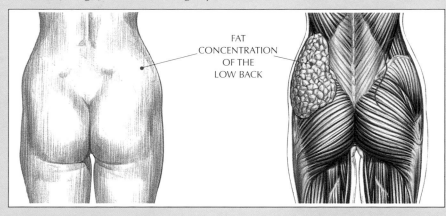

FAT CONCENTRATION OF THE LOW BACK

3. BELOW THE TROCHANTER, OR "RIDING BREECHES"

Frequently found in Mediterranean women, this concentration can be quite bulky. Located on the superior part of the lateral thigh just below the depression of the greater trochanter, it blends with the fatty tissue of the anterior surface of the thigh and, at the posterior, with that of the buttocks. When there is a lot of fat in this area we often observe many more or less deep depressions on the surface of the skin, referred to as a "pitted" or "cottage cheese" surface. This is due to inelastic fibrous tracts that, like little cables, connect the deep surface of the skin at the level of the depressions to the enveloping aponeurosis of the muscle, with the adipose tissue creating bumps or bulges in between (a quiltlike phenomenon).

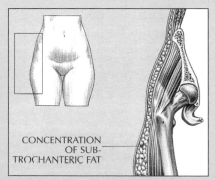

CONCENTRATION OF SUB-TROCHANTERIC FAT

4. BETWEEN THE THIGHS

Relatively common in women, fat in this location plays an important aesthetic role in that it fills the space between the two thighs; it is often more noticeable in women than in men.

5. AROUND THE NAVEL

As in the subtrochanteric location, the periumbilical concentration is one of the rare fat deposits that is also found in thin women.

6. PUBIS

This triangular concentration is known as the "mount of Venus." It protects the symphysis pubis from blows.

7. KNEE

In women, the knee is often a location of fat concentration, especially on the medial region.

8. POSTERIOR-MEDIAL PART OF THE UPPER ARM

Especially developed in women, this concentration, besides its energetic role, protects the superficial nerves and arteries in the medial and superior area of the arm.

9. BREASTS

The breast is composed of fat enclosing the mammary glands, the whole being held together by a web of connective tissue resting on the pectoralis major. Note that men also have glands and mammary fat (atrophied).

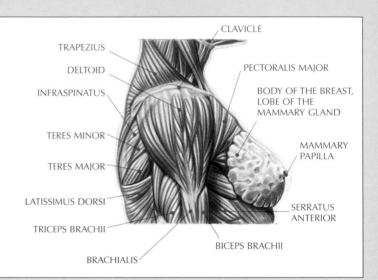

CELLULITE

Fat is made up of cells called *adipocytes*, whose main function is to stockpile energy reserves. Thus these cells accumulate energy in the form of lipids, which they release back to the body on demand. These adipocytes are present as small accumulations of fat that are walled off by fibrous connective tissue. These fat nodules spread in clusters between the dermis (the tissue that makes up the deep layer of the skin) and the muscles. When the adipocytes accumulate more energy than is consumed, they tend to grow considerably in size and fat begins to accumulate.

On the surface of the skin of the buttocks and the hips in women, we often observe multiple, more or less deep depressions that are commonly called "cottage cheese." This appearance is caused by inelastic fibrous tracts in these areas, which, like little cables, attach the envelope of the muscles to the deep surface of the skin at the depressions, with the fatty tissue bulging in between (like a quilt).

This characteristic has an important effect in women: When the body consumes fewer calories than it absorbs, the fat reserves increase. This subcutaneous fat, or cellulite, is compartmentalized by a fibrous connective tissue net. When this net is compressed, the lymphatics and blood vessels that run through the area are also compressed, the organic exchanges are slowed down, and the blood does not readily reach these fatty quilted areas to remove the stockpiled fatty acids. It is therefore easy to understand that the localized fat becomes difficult for the body to remove and that even intensive training may not remove it completely. For example, it is not unusual for a woman on a strict diet to lose weight, lose her breasts . . . but keep her hips.

Hormonal causes: Hormones also play a role in the appearance of cellulite and its increase. In fact, in women hormonal variations—and especially the excessive amounts of estrogen during the menstrual cycle or during pregnancy—favor subcutaneous water retention. This water retention associated with fat compresses the lymphatic and blood vessels, which slows down circulation and makes the subcutaneous energetic reserves more difficult for the organism to mobilize.

These systems for protecting and storing fat in women have evolved to maintain fat reserves that are available during the last six months of pregnancy and for breastfeeding in times of scarcity.

BUTTOCKS

1. STATIC FORWARD LUNGES
2. FORWARD LUNGES WITH A BAR
3. FORWARD LUNGES WITH A ROD
4. FORWARD LUNGES WITH DUMBBELLS
5. BENCH STEPS
6. STANDING HIP ABDUCTIONS
7. STANDING HIP ABDUCTIONS WITH AN ELASTIC BAND
8. CABLE HIP ABDUCTIONS
9. STANDING MACHINE HIP ABDUCTIONS
10. FLOOR HIP ABDUCTIONS WITH AN ELASTIC BAND
11. FLOOR HIP ABDUCTIONS
12. SEATED MACHINE HIP ABDUCTIONS
13. LATERAL THIGH RAISES ON THE FLOOR
14. MACHINE HIP EXTENSIONS
15. STANDING HIP EXTENSIONS
16. FLOOR HIP EXTENSIONS
17. MACHINE HIP EXTENSIONS LYING DOWN
18. HIP EXTENSIONS WITH A LOW PULLEY
19. FLOOR HIP EXTENSIONS WITH AN ELASTIC BAND
20. HIP EXTENSIONS ON A BENCH
21. PRONE HIP EXTENSIONS
22. STANDING HIP EXTENSIONS WITH AN ELASTIC BAND
23. PELVIC RAISES OFF THE FLOOR
24. PELVIC RAISES ON ONE LEG
25. PELVIC RAISES OFF A BENCH
26. POSTERIOR PELVIC TILTS
27. SMALL LATERAL THIGH FLEXIONS

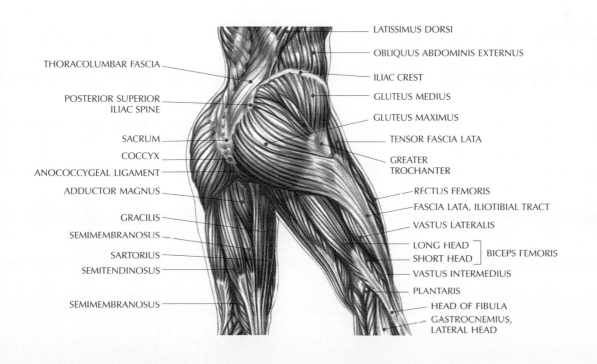

THORACOLUMBAR FASCIA

POSTERIOR SUPERIOR ILIAC SPINE

SACRUM

COCCYX

ANOCOCCYGEAL LIGAMENT

ADDUCTOR MAGNUS

GRACILIS

SEMIMEMBRANOSUS

SARTORIUS

SEMITENDINOSUS

SEMIMEMBRANOSUS

LATISSIMUS DORSI

OBLIQUUS ABDOMINIS EXTERNUS

ILIAC CREST

GLUTEUS MEDIUS

GLUTEUS MAXIMUS

TENSOR FASCIA LATA

GREATER TROCHANTER

RECTUS FEMORIS

FASCIA LATA, ILIOTIBIAL TRACT

VASTUS LATERALIS

LONG HEAD
SHORT HEAD } BICEPS FEMORIS

VASTUS INTERMEDIUS

PLANTARIS

HEAD OF FIBULA

GASTROCNEMIUS, LATERAL HEAD

THE GLUTEAL DELTOID

The deltoid of the shoulder and the gluteal deltoid both act to move an extremity through numerous planes in space.

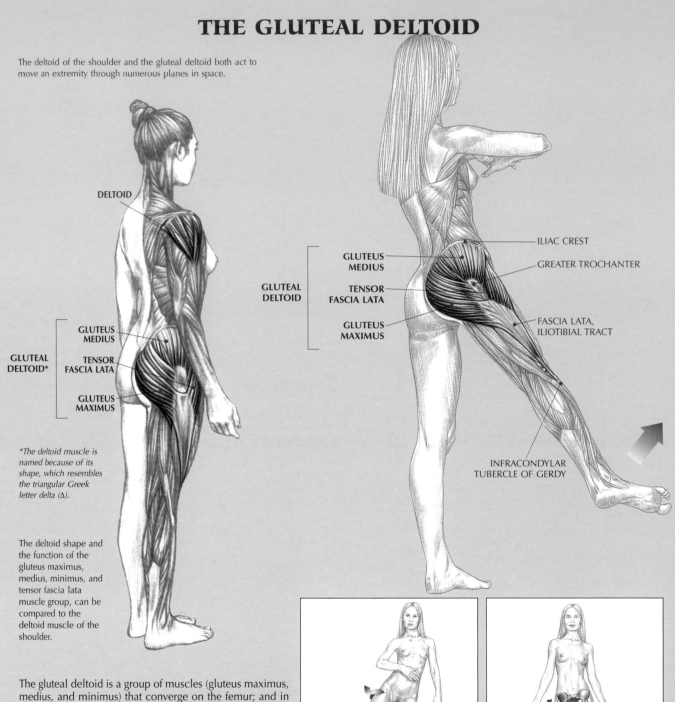

DELTOID

GLUTEUS
MEDIUS

GLUTEAL
DELTOID*

TENSOR
FASCIA LATA

GLUTEUS
MAXIMUS

The deltoid muscle is named because of its shape, which resembles the triangular Greek letter delta (Δ).

The deltoid shape and the function of the gluteus maximus, medius, minimus, and tensor fascia lata muscle group, can be compared to the deltoid muscle of the shoulder.

GLUTEAL
DELTOID

GLUTEUS
MEDIUS

TENSOR
FASCIA LATA

GLUTEUS
MAXIMUS

ILIAC CREST

GREATER TROCHANTER

FASCIA LATA,
ILIOTIBIAL TRACT

INFRACONDYLAR
TUBERCLE OF GERDY

The gluteal deltoid is a group of muscles (gluteus maximus, medius, and minimus) that converge on the femur; and in the superficial plane, converge on the fascia lata or iliotibial tract* (superficial portion of the gluteus maximus and tensor fascia lata muscles). When the gluteal deltoid muscle group work together as synergists they abduct the hip. Just like its counterpart at the shoulder—the deltoid, the main muscle of the shoulder—the gluteal deltoid acts to move the lower extremity through numerous planes in space.

The fascia lata or iliotibial tract of the thigh is a thickening of the aponeurosis, which wraps and contains the muscles of the thigh. This thickening attaches inferiorly to the tibia at the level of Gerdy's tubercle.

The gluteus minimus and the anterior fibers of the gluteus medius engage the femur in internal flexion-rotation and abduction.

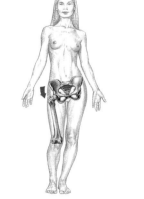

When the femur is fixed, the gluteal deltoid tilts the pelvis laterally.

OBLIQUUS ABDOMINIS EXTERNUS

LATISSIMUS DORSI

ILIOPSOAS

GLUTEUS MEDIUS

GLUTEUS MAXIMUS

ADDUCTOR MAGNUS

SEMIMEMBRANOSUS

SEMITENDINOSUS

BICEPS FEMORIS

GRACILIS

SARTORIUS

SOLEUS

TRICEPS SURAE

GASTROCNEMIUS, MEDIAL HEAD

GASTROCNEMIUS, LATERAL HEAD

VASTUS MEDIALIS

RECTUS FEMORIS

RECTUS FEMORIS
VASTUS LATERALIS **QUADRICEPS**
VASTUS INTERMEDIUS

PATELLA

FASCIA LATA, ILIOTIBIAL TRACT

SHORT HEAD
LONG HEAD **BICEPS FEMORIS**

PERONEUS LONGUS

EXTENSOR DIGITORUM COMMUNIS

TIBIALIS ANTERIOR

PERONEUS BREVIS

INITIAL POSITION

Stand with your knees slightly flexed, one foot in front of the other, with your feet slightly farther apart than in a normal step; rest your hands on the front thigh. Keep your back straight, chest forward. Inhale and flex the forward thigh until it is horizontal. Extend it to return to the initial position. Exhale at the end of the movement.

- The farther the feet are apart the more the gluteus maximus is worked.
- The closer the feet are together the more the quadriceps are worked.

For better results work this movement in alternating long series on one side and then the other; you must feel the muscle working.

Note

As in all anterior lunge positions, this is a good stretch for the rectus muscle of the thigh and the iliopsoas muscle of the posterior leg. The position with the hands on the thighs allows the exercise to be performed with greater stability.

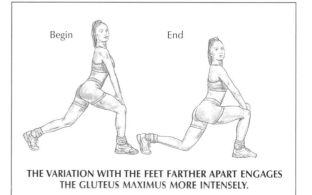

Begin   End

THE VARIATION WITH THE FEET FARTHER APART ENGAGES THE GLUTEUS MAXIMUS MORE INTENSELY.

2 FORWARD LUNGES WITH A BAR

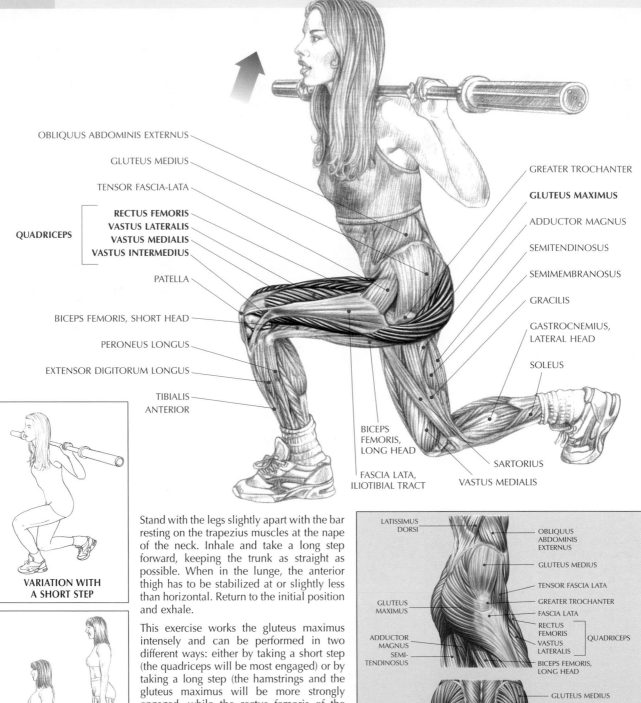

OBLIQUUS ABDOMINIS EXTERNUS

GLUTEUS MEDIUS

TENSOR FASCIA-LATA

RECTUS FEMORIS
VASTUS LATERALIS
QUADRICEPS **VASTUS MEDIALIS**
VASTUS INTERMEDIUS

PATELLA

BICEPS FEMORIS, SHORT HEAD

PERONEUS LONGUS

EXTENSOR DIGITORUM LONGUS

TIBIALIS ANTERIOR

BICEPS FEMORIS, LONG HEAD

FASCIA LATA, ILIOTIBIAL TRACT

GREATER TROCHANTER

GLUTEUS MAXIMUS

ADDUCTOR MAGNUS

SEMITENDINOSUS

SEMIMEMBRANOSUS

GRACILIS

GASTROCNEMIUS, LATERAL HEAD

SOLEUS

SARTORIUS

VASTUS MEDIALIS

VARIATION WITH A SHORT STEP

VARIATION WITH DUMBBELLS

Stand with the legs slightly apart with the bar resting on the trapezius muscles at the nape of the neck. Inhale and take a long step forward, keeping the trunk as straight as possible. When in the lunge, the anterior thigh has to be stabilized at or slightly less than horizontal. Return to the initial position and exhale.

This exercise works the gluteus maximus intensely and can be performed in two different ways: either by taking a short step (the quadriceps will be most engaged) or by taking a long step (the hamstrings and the gluteus maximus will be more strongly engaged, while the rectus femoris of the posterior thigh and the iliopsoas of the posterior leg will be stretched).

Note
Because most of the weight will be on the anterior leg and the movement requires a good sense of balance, it is recommended to begin with very light weights.

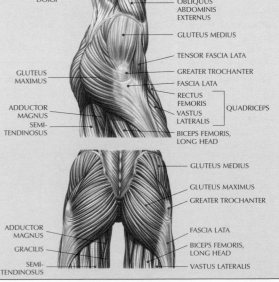

LATISSIMUS DORSI

GLUTEUS MAXIMUS

ADDUCTOR MAGNUS

SEMI-TENDINOSUS

OBLIQUUS ABDOMINIS EXTERNUS

GLUTEUS MEDIUS

TENSOR FASCIA LATA

GREATER TROCHANTER

FASCIA LATA

RECTUS FEMORIS
VASTUS LATERALIS QUADRICEPS

BICEPS FEMORIS, LONG HEAD

GLUTEUS MEDIUS

GLUTEUS MAXIMUS

GREATER TROCHANTER

FASCIA LATA

BICEPS FEMORIS, LONG HEAD

VASTUS LATERALIS

ADDUCTOR MAGNUS

GRACILIS

SEMI-TENDINOSUS

FORWARD LUNGES WITH A ROD

3

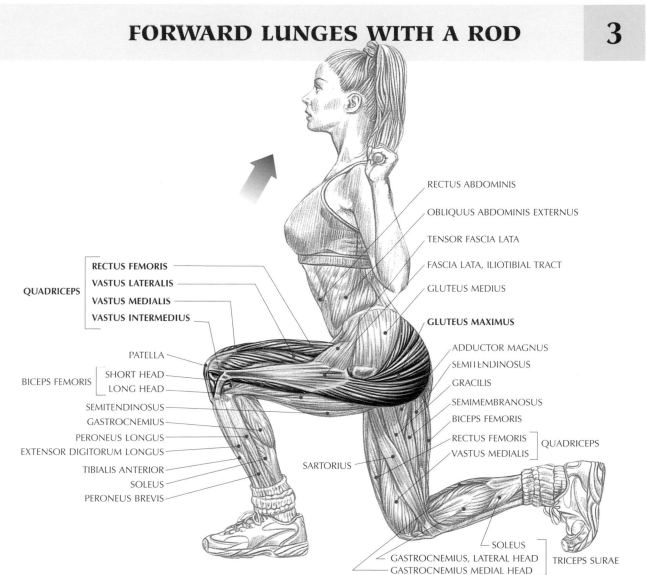

RECTUS ABDOMINIS

OBLIQUUS ABDOMINIS EXTERNUS

TENSOR FASCIA LATA

FASCIA LATA, ILIOTIBIAL TRACT

GLUTEUS MEDIUS

GLUTEUS MAXIMUS

ADDUCTOR MAGNUS

SEMITENDINOSUS

GRACILIS

SEMIMEMBRANOSUS

BICEPS FEMORIS

RECTUS FEMORIS — QUADRICEPS

VASTUS MEDIALIS

SARTORIUS

SOLEUS

GASTROCNEMIUS, LATERAL HEAD — TRICEPS SURAE

GASTROCNEMIUS MEDIAL HEAD

QUADRICEPS
RECTUS FEMORIS
VASTUS LATERALIS
VASTUS MEDIALIS
VASTUS INTERMEDIUS

PATELLA

BICEPS FEMORIS
SHORT HEAD
LONG HEAD

SEMITENDINOSUS
GASTROCNEMIUS
PERONEUS LONGUS
EXTENSOR DIGITORUM LONGUS
TIBIALIS ANTERIOR
SOLEUS
PERONEUS BREVIS

Stand with legs slightly apart and with the rod resting on the trapezius muscles at the nape of the neck. Inhale and take a big step forward, keeping the chest as straight as possible. When the forward thigh reaches horizontal or slightly below, perform a tonic extension to return it to the initial position. Exhale on return to standing.

This exercise works mainly on the gluteus maximus as well as the quadriceps. Taking a small step will engage the quadriceps more intensely. This is an excellent exercise for developing a good sense of balance and to increase strength before working with weights. Furthermore, performing the movement with a big step is a good stretch for the iliopsoas and the rectus femoris of the posterior leg. Because this exercise combines working muscles and stretching them, it has become part of the warm-up routine for many athletes.

It is possible to perform the lunges by alternating left and right during the same series or to perform them first on one side and then the other.

Note

The weight of the body mostly rests on one leg for most of the exercise, so it is recommended that people with fragile knees perform the lunges carefully.

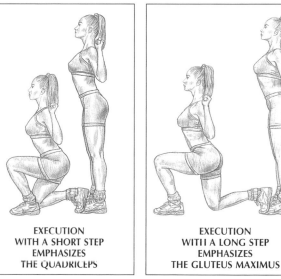

EXECUTION
WITH A SHORT STEP
EMPHASIZES
THE QUADRICEPS

EXECUTION
WITH A LONG STEP
EMPHASIZES
THE GLUTEUS MAXIMUS

4 FORWARD LUNGES WITH DUMBBELLS

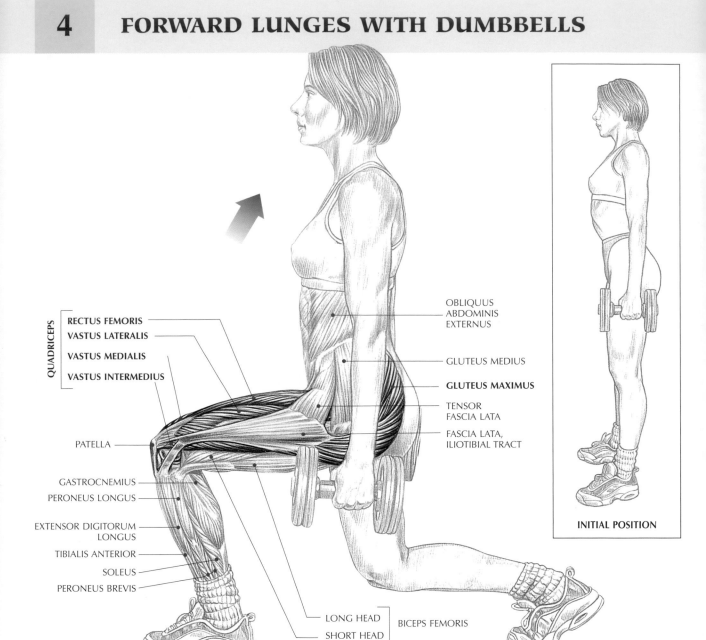

QUADRICEPS
- **RECTUS FEMORIS**
- **VASTUS LATERALIS**
- **VASTUS MEDIALIS**
- **VASTUS INTERMEDIUS**

OBLIQUUS ABDOMINIS EXTERNUS

GLUTEUS MEDIUS

GLUTEUS MAXIMUS

TENSOR FASCIA LATA

FASCIA LATA, ILIOTIBIAL TRACT

PATELLA

GASTROCNEMIUS

PERONEUS LONGUS

EXTENSOR DIGITORUM LONGUS

TIBIALIS ANTERIOR

SOLEUS

PERONEUS BREVIS

LONG HEAD
SHORT HEAD
BICEPS FEMORIS

INITIAL POSITION

Stand with the legs slightly apart and a dumbbell in each hand. Inhale and take a big step forward, keeping the chest as straight as possible. When the front thigh reaches horizontal or slightly below horizontal, return to the initial position, maintaining it in tonic extension. Exhale at the end of the movement.

This exercise mainly works the gluteus maximus and quadriceps.

Note
All the weight rests on the anterior leg at some point, and this movement requires a good sense of balance. To protect the knee, it is recommended that beginners start with light weights.

Variations
- The bigger the step the more the gluteus maximus of the front leg will be engaged and the more the iliopsoas and rectus femoris of the back leg will be stretched.
- The smaller the step the more the quadriceps muscles of the front leg will be engaged.

It is possible to perform a complete series on one side and then on the other or to alternate between left and right during the same series.

BENCH STEPS

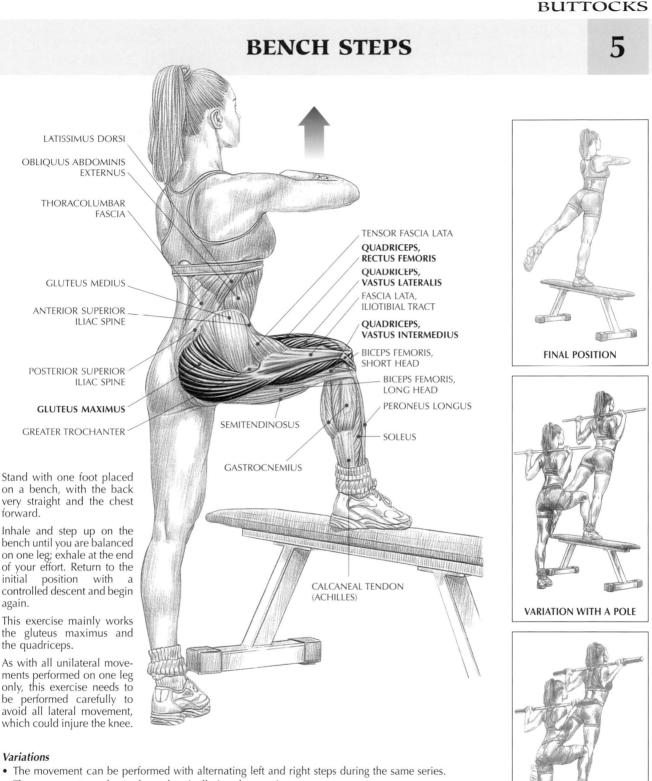

LATISSIMUS DORSI

OBLIQUUS ABDOMINIS EXTERNUS

THORACOLUMBAR FASCIA

GLUTEUS MEDIUS

ANTERIOR SUPERIOR ILIAC SPINE

POSTERIOR SUPERIOR ILIAC SPINE

GLUTEUS MAXIMUS

GREATER TROCHANTER

SEMITENDINOSUS

GASTROCNEMIUS

TENSOR FASCIA LATA

QUADRICEPS, RECTUS FEMORIS

QUADRICEPS, VASTUS LATERALIS

FASCIA LATA, ILIOTIBIAL TRACT

QUADRICEPS, VASTUS INTERMEDIUS

BICEPS FEMORIS, SHORT HEAD

BICEPS FEMORIS, LONG HEAD

PERONEUS LONGUS

SOLEUS

CALCANEAL TENDON (ACHILLES)

FINAL POSITION

VARIATION WITH A POLE

VARIATION WITH A BAR

Stand with one foot placed on a bench, with the back very straight and the chest forward.

Inhale and step up on the bench until you are balanced on one leg; exhale at the end of your effort. Return to the initial position with a controlled descent and begin again.

This exercise mainly works the gluteus maximus and the quadriceps.

As with all unilateral movements performed on one leg only, this exercise needs to be performed carefully to avoid all lateral movement, which could injure the knee.

Variations

- The movement can be performed with alternating left and right steps during the same series.
- The movement can be performed tonically in a long series.
- Stepping up on the bench without using the leg on the ground will work the gluteus maximus harder.
- Using a pole on the shoulders to avoid thrusting with the arms will make the leg work harder.
- The movement can be performed with a bar on the shoulders (favored by 100-, 200- and 400-meter sprinters). Although very effective for working the gluteals, the quadriceps, and balance, this last variation needs to be executed very carefully (especially on the return to the ground) to protect the knee and the lumbar spine. This kind of bench step is contraindicated for people with back or knee problems.

6 STANDING HIP ABDUCTIONS

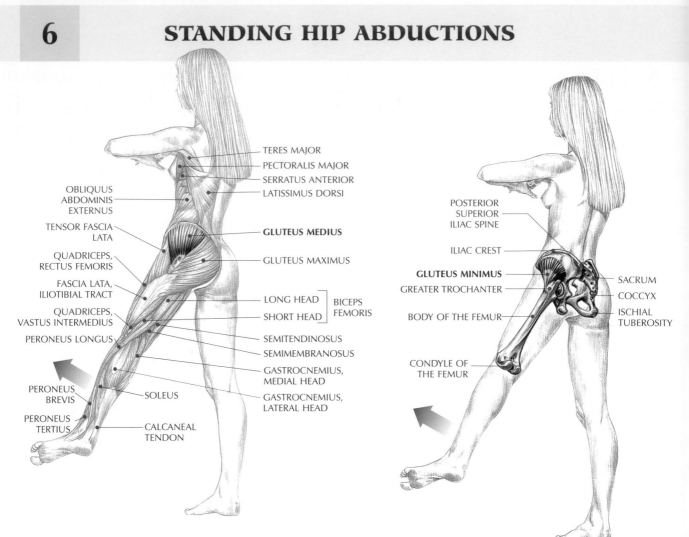

TERES MAJOR
PECTORALIS MAJOR
SERRATUS ANTERIOR
LATISSIMUS DORSI

OBLIQUUS ABDOMINIS EXTERNUS

TENSOR FASCIA LATA

GLUTEUS MEDIUS

QUADRICEPS, RECTUS FEMORIS

GLUTEUS MAXIMUS

FASCIA LATA, ILIOTIBIAL TRACT

QUADRICEPS, VASTUS INTERMEDIUS

LONG HEAD } BICEPS
SHORT HEAD } FEMORIS

PERONEUS LONGUS

SEMITENDINOSUS
SEMIMEMBRANOSUS

GASTROCNEMIUS, MEDIAL HEAD

PERONEUS BREVIS

SOLEUS

GASTROCNEMIUS, LATERAL HEAD

PERONEUS TERTIUS

CALCANEAL TENDON

POSTERIOR SUPERIOR ILIAC SPINE

ILIAC CREST

GLUTEUS MINIMUS
GREATER TROCHANTER

SACRUM
COCCYX

BODY OF THE FEMUR

ISCHIAL TUBEROSITY

CONDYLE OF THE FEMUR

Stand on one leg with the arms crossed in front, or for more stability with one hand resting on a stable support.

Raise the leg laterally as high as possible. Slowly return to the initial position and begin again.

This exercise, which engages the gluteal deltoid, mainly works the gluteus medius and the deeper gluteus minimus.

Note
- By raising the leg slightly more to the front, you will work the tensor fascia lata muscle more intensely.
- By raising the leg slightly more to the back, you will work the superior fibers of the gluteus maximus more intensely.

  Abduction of the hip is limited at the osseous level by the abutment of the neck of the femur against the border of the acetabulum of the os coxa (pelvis); it is useless to try to raise the leg to horizontal.

  Doing long series until you feel a burn will produce the best results.

Variations
- For greater intensity use ankle weights or an elastic band.
- For more stability perform the movement using a staff for support.

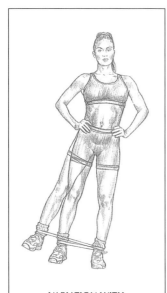

VARIATION WITH AN ELASTIC BAND

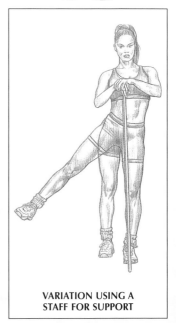

VARIATION USING A STAFF FOR SUPPORT

STANDING HIP ABDUCTIONS
WITH AN ELASTIC BAND

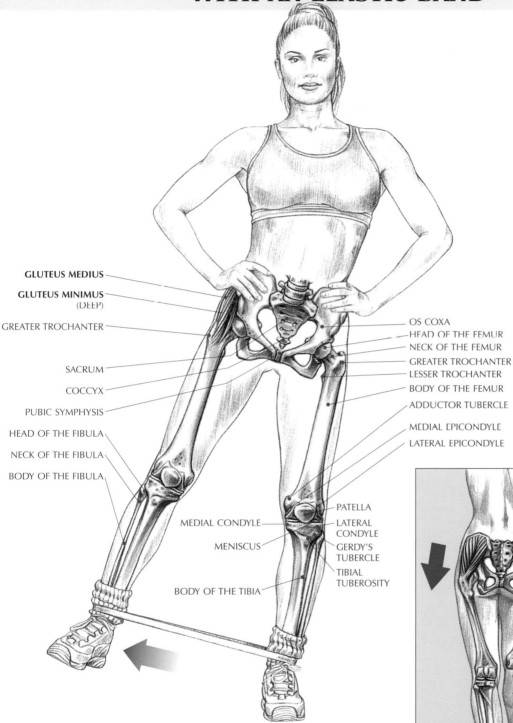

GLUTEUS MEDIUS

GLUTEUS MINIMUS
(DEEP)

GREATER TROCHANTER

SACRUM

COCCYX

PUBIC SYMPHYSIS

HEAD OF THE FIBULA

NECK OF THE FIBULA

BODY OF THE FIBULA

MEDIAL CONDYLE

MENISCUS

BODY OF THE TIBIA

OS COXA

HEAD OF THE FEMUR

NECK OF THE FEMUR

GREATER TROCHANTER

LESSER TROCHANTER

BODY OF THE FEMUR

ADDUCTOR TUBERCLE

MEDIAL EPICONDYLE

LATERAL EPICONDYLE

PATELLA

LATERAL CONDYLE

GERDY'S TUBERCLE

TIBIAL TUBEROSITY

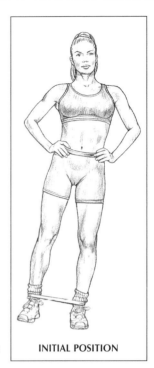

INITIAL POSITION

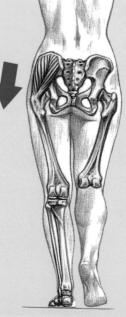

ROLE OF GLUTEUS MEDIUS AND MINIMUS IN GAIT

Besides their role in hip abduction, the gluteus medius and minimus play an important role in gait as they stabilize the pelvis, preventing it from tilting sideways when on one foot.

Stand on one leg with an elastic band around the ankles. Perform small hip abductions.

As with all exercises using an elastic band, you only obtain good results with long series. By doubling the elastic band, you increase the intensity of the effort but decrease the amplitude of the movement. This exercise works the gluteus medius and the deeper gluteus minimus.

8 CABLE HIP ABDUCTIONS

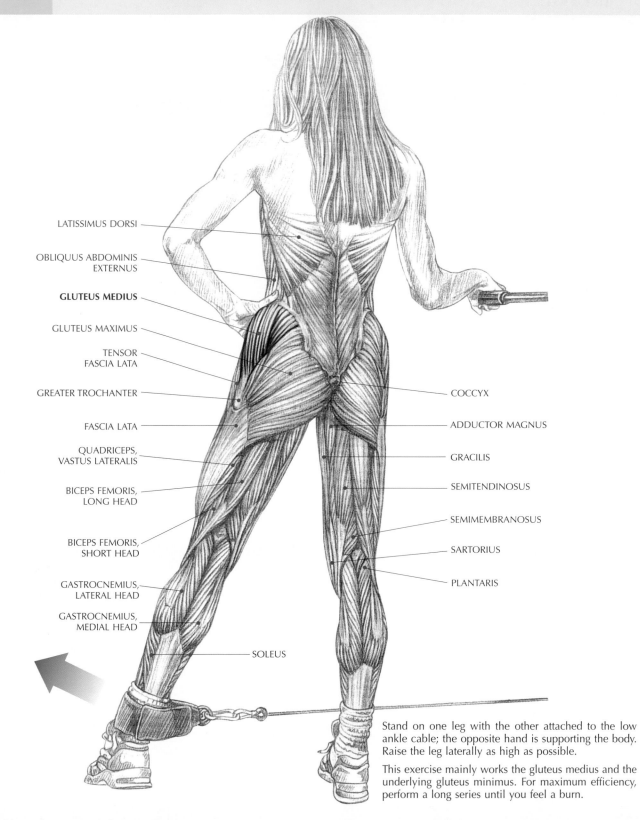

LATISSIMUS DORSI

OBLIQUUS ABDOMINIS EXTERNUS

GLUTEUS MEDIUS

GLUTEUS MAXIMUS

TENSOR FASCIA LATA

GREATER TROCHANTER

FASCIA LATA

QUADRICEPS, VASTUS LATERALIS

BICEPS FEMORIS, LONG HEAD

BICEPS FEMORIS, SHORT HEAD

GASTROCNEMIUS, LATERAL HEAD

GASTROCNEMIUS, MEDIAL HEAD

SOLEUS

COCCYX

ADDUCTOR MAGNUS

GRACILIS

SEMITENDINOSUS

SEMIMEMBRANOSUS

SARTORIUS

PLANTARIS

Stand on one leg with the other attached to the low ankle cable; the opposite hand is supporting the body. Raise the leg laterally as high as possible.

This exercise mainly works the gluteus medius and the underlying gluteus minimus. For maximum efficiency, perform a long series until you feel a burn.

INDIVIDUAL VARIATIONS IN HIP MOBILITY

Aside from individual variations of muscle flexibility and ligament laxity, it is above all the shape of the bones at the coxo-femoral joint that mainly accounts for variations in hip mobility.

It is mainly with hip abduction that the shape of the bone plays an important role.

Example

- An almost horizontal femoral neck (coxa vara), associated with a more developed superior border of the acetabulum, limits abduction movements.
- A more vertical femoral neck (coxa valga), associated with a less developed superior border of the acetabulum, facilitates abduction.

Therefore, it is useless to try to raise the hip higher than what the morphology will allow.

If hip abduction is forced, the neck of the femur will butt against the border of the acetabulum and the pelvis will compensate by tilting onto the opposite femoral head. Furthermore, performing a series of forced abductions may eventually lead to microtrauma, which will lead to excessive development of the superior border of the acetabulum, limiting the mobility of the hip as well as risking painful inflammation.

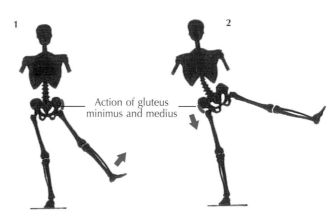

Action of gluteus minimus and medius

1. Hip abduction (limited by the neck of the femur butting against the border of the acetabulum).
2. Forced abduction of the hip (tilting of the pelvis onto the opposite femoral head).

THE DIFFERENT OSSEOUS HIP MORPHOLOGIES

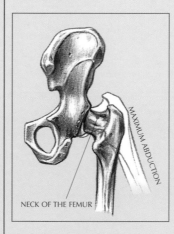

An almost horizontal femoral neck, called **coxa vara**, limits hip abduction as it butts up against the superior border of the acetabulum.

NECK OF THE FEMUR

MAXIMUM ABDUCTION

A close to vertical femoral neck, called a **coxa valga**, facilitates greater hip abduction.

MAXIMUM ABDUCTION

NECK OF THE FEMUR

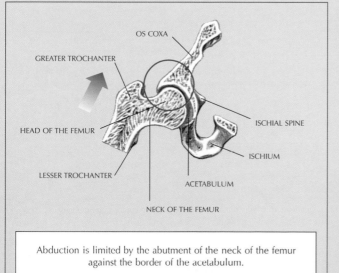

OS COXA

GREATER TROCHANTER

HEAD OF THE FEMUR

LESSER TROCHANTER

ISCHIAL SPINE

ISCHIUM

ACETABULUM

NECK OF THE FEMUR

Abduction is limited by the abutment of the neck of the femur against the border of the acetabulum.

STANDING MACHINE HIP ABDUCTIONS

9

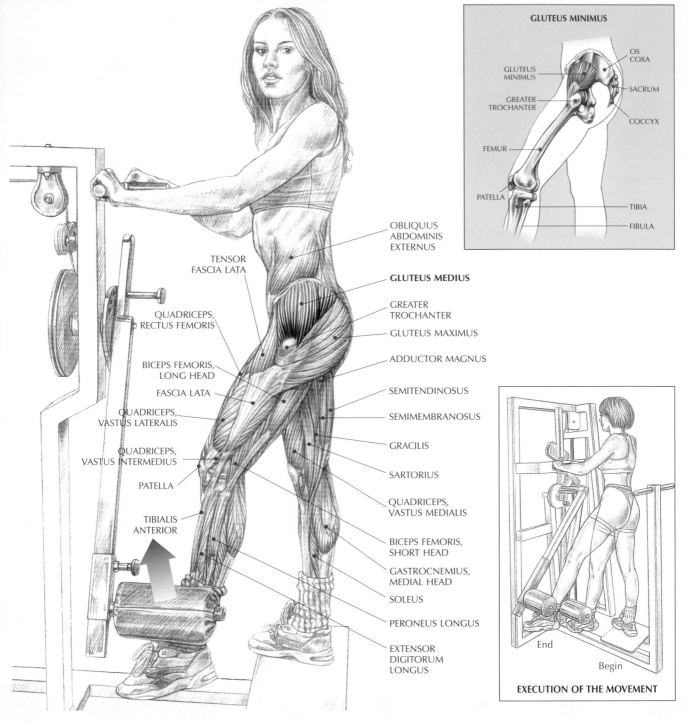

GLUTEUS MINIMUS

GLUTEUS MINIMUS

OS COXA

SACRUM

GREATER TROCHANTER

COCCYX

FEMUR

PATELLA

TIBIA

FIBULA

OBLIQUUS ABDOMINIS EXTERNUS

TENSOR FASCIA LATA

GLUTEUS MEDIUS

GREATER TROCHANTER

QUADRICEPS, RECTUS FEMORIS

GLUTEUS MAXIMUS

ADDUCTOR MAGNUS

BICEPS FEMORIS, LONG HEAD

SEMITENDINOSUS

FASCIA LATA

SEMIMEMBRANOSUS

QUADRICEPS, VASTUS LATERALIS

GRACILIS

QUADRICEPS, VASTUS INTERMEDIUS

SARTORIUS

PATELLA

QUADRICEPS, VASTUS MEDIALIS

TIBIALIS ANTERIOR

BICEPS FEMORIS, SHORT HEAD

GASTROCNEMIUS, MEDIAL HEAD

SOLEUS

PERONEUS LONGUS

EXTENSOR DIGITORUM LONGUS

End

Begin

EXECUTION OF THE MOVEMENT

Stand on one leg at the machine, with the pad placed against the outside of the opposite lower leg, below the knee joint.

Raise the leg laterally as high as possible and slowly return it to the initial position. Note that abduction is soon limited by the fact that the neck of the femur quickly butts against the border of the acetabulum.

This exercise is excellent for developing the gluteus medius and underlying gluteus minimus, which functions the as the anterior fibers of the gluteus medius. For best results, work in long series.

FLOOR HIP ABDUCTIONS WITH AN ELASTIC BAND

10

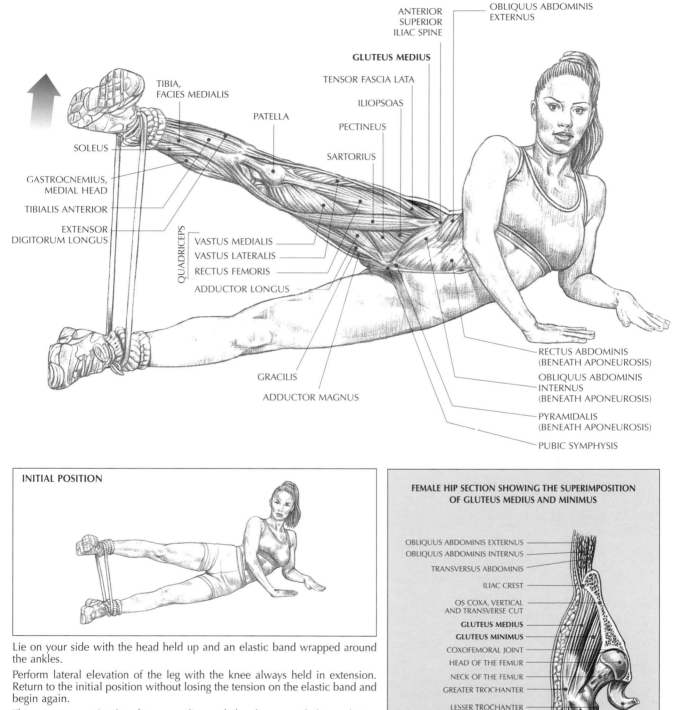

SOLEUS

GASTROCNEMIUS, MEDIAL HEAD

TIBIALIS ANTERIOR

EXTENSOR DIGITORUM LONGUS

TIBIA, FACIES MEDIALIS

PATELLA

QUADRICEPS

VASTUS MEDIALIS

VASTUS LATERALIS

RECTUS FEMORIS

ADDUCTOR LONGUS

GRACILIS

ADDUCTOR MAGNUS

ANTERIOR SUPERIOR ILIAC SPINE

GLUTEUS MEDIUS

TENSOR FASCIA LATA

ILIOPSOAS

PECTINEUS

SARTORIUS

OBLIQUUS ABDOMINIS EXTERNUS

RECTUS ABDOMINIS (BENEATH APONEUROSIS)

OBLIQUUS ABDOMINIS INTERNUS (BENEATH APONEUROSIS)

PYRAMIDALIS (BENEATH APONEUROSIS)

PUBIC SYMPHYSIS

INITIAL POSITION

Lie on your side with the head held up and an elastic band wrapped around the ankles.

Perform lateral elevation of the leg with the knee always held in extension. Return to the initial position without losing the tension on the elastic band and begin again.

This exercise works the gluteus medius and the deeper underlying gluteus minimus, main muscles of the curve of the thigh.

Long series produce better results.

Note

For greater intensity it is possible to perform the movement with two elastic bands around the ankles.

FEMALE HIP SECTION SHOWING THE SUPERIMPOSITION OF GLUTEUS MEDIUS AND MINIMUS

OBLIQUUS ABDOMINIS EXTERNUS

OBLIQUUS ABDOMINIS INTERNUS

TRANSVERSUS ABDOMINIS

ILIAC CREST

OS COXA, VERTICAL AND TRANSVERSE CUT

GLUTEUS MEDIUS

GLUTEUS MINIMUS

COXOFEMORAL JOINT

HEAD OF THE FEMUR

NECK OF THE FEMUR

GREATER TROCHANTER

LESSER TROCHANTER

FEMUR

QUADRICEPS, VASTUS LATERALIS

SUBCUTANEOUS LAYER OF ADIPOSE PANICULUS

RAMUS OF THE ISCHIUM

11 FLOOR HIP ABDUCTIONS

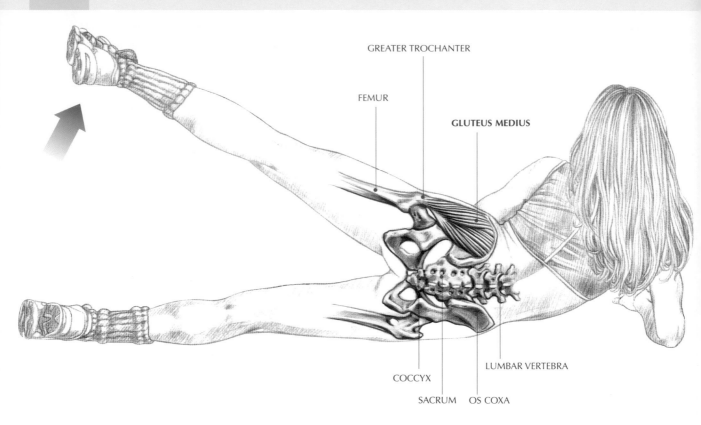

GREATER TROCHANTER

FEMUR

GLUTEUS MEDIUS

COCCYX

SACRUM   OS COXA

LUMBAR VERTEBRA

EXECUTION OF THE MOVEMENT

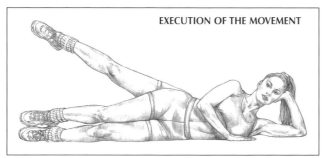

Maintain the head up while lying on the side.

Perform a lateral leg raise, with the knee always in extension, so that abduction is no greater than 70 degrees.

This exercise works the gluteus medius and minimus. It can be performed with greater or lesser amplitude. You may also maintain a few seconds of isometric contraction at the end of the abduction.

The leg may be raised slightly anterior or posterior or vertically. For more efficiency you may use ankle weights or eventually an elastic band or low ankle cable.

THE 3 WAYS OF RAISING THE LEG

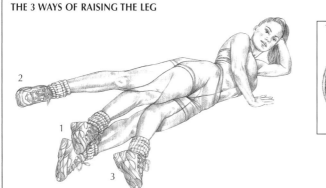

SOLICITED ZONES

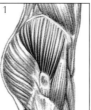 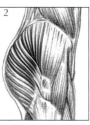 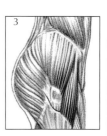

1. Leg raised vertically

2. Leg raised slightly posterior

3. Leg raised slightly anterior

SEATED MACHINE HIP ABDUCTIONS

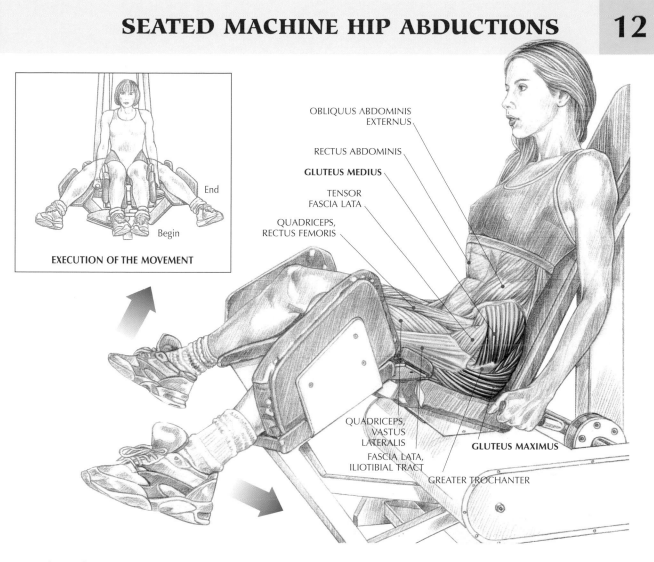

EXECUTION OF THE MOVEMENT

End

Begin

OBLIQUUS ABDOMINIS EXTERNUS

RECTUS ABDOMINIS

GLUTEUS MEDIUS

TENSOR FASCIA LATA

QUADRICEPS, RECTUS FEMORIS

QUADRICEPS, VASTUS LATERALIS

FASCIA LATA, ILIOTIBIAL TRACT

GLUTEUS MAXIMUS

GREATER TROCHANTER

Sit on the machine. Open the thighs as wide as possible. The more the back of the machine is tilted back, the more the gluteus medius muscles are solicited; the closer the back of the machine is to vertical the more the superior portion of the gluteus maximus muscles will be worked. Ideally you will vary the angle of the torso during the same series by leaning more or less forward.

Example

Ten repetitions with the torso leaning back followed by 10 repetitions with the torso leaning forward. This exercise is excellent for women as it firms up the upper part of the hips while shaping the curve of the thigh, which helps create the appearance of a thinner waistline.

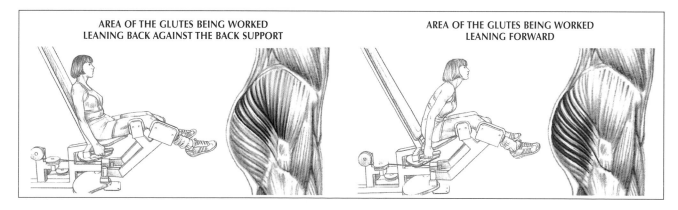

AREA OF THE GLUTES BEING WORKED LEANING BACK AGAINST THE BACK SUPPORT

AREA OF THE GLUTES BEING WORKED LEANING FORWARD

13   LATERAL THIGH RAISES
ON THE FLOOR

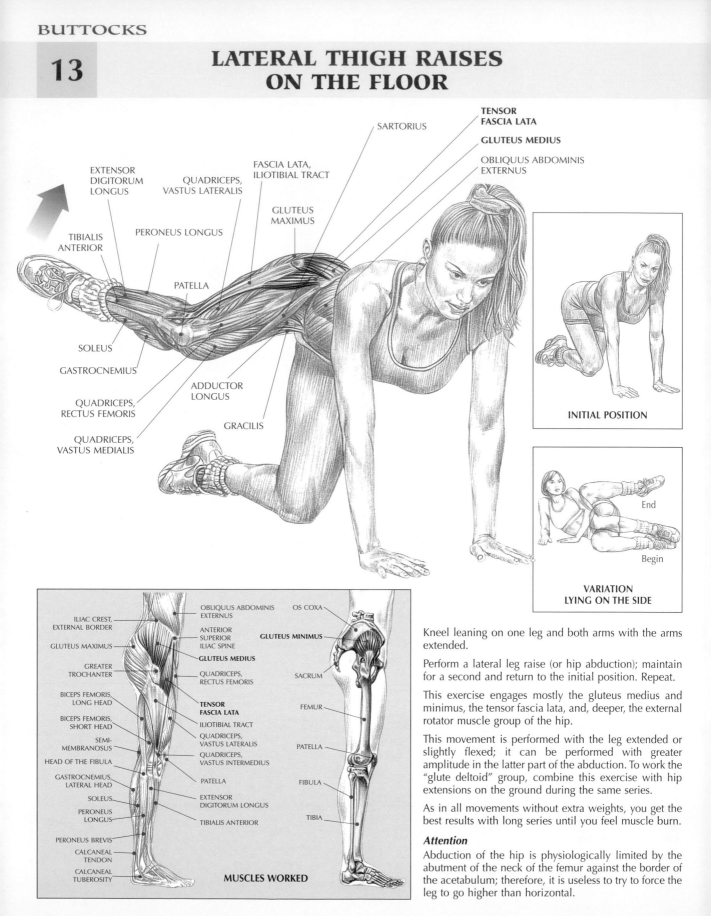

SARTORIUS

TENSOR
FASCIA LATA

GLUTEUS MEDIUS

OBLIQUUS ABDOMINIS
EXTERNUS

FASCIA LATA,
ILIOTIBIAL TRACT

EXTENSOR
DIGITORUM
LONGUS

QUADRICEPS,
VASTUS LATERALIS

GLUTEUS
MAXIMUS

TIBIALIS
ANTERIOR

PERONEUS LONGUS

PATELLA

SOLEUS

GASTROCNEMIUS

QUADRICEPS,
RECTUS FEMORIS

ADDUCTOR
LONGUS

GRACILIS

QUADRICEPS,
VASTUS MEDIALIS

INITIAL POSITION

End

Begin

**VARIATION
LYING ON THE SIDE**

MUSCLES WORKED

ILIAC CREST,
EXTERNAL BORDER

OBLIQUUS ABDOMINIS
EXTERNUS

OS COXA

GLUTEUS MAXIMUS

ANTERIOR
SUPERIOR
ILIAC SPINE

GLUTEUS MINIMUS

GREATER
TROCHANTER

GLUTEUS MEDIUS

SACRUM

QUADRICEPS,
RECTUS FEMORIS

BICEPS FEMORIS,
LONG HEAD

TENSOR
FASCIA LATA

FEMUR

BICEPS FEMORIS,
SHORT HEAD

ILIOTIBIAL TRACT

SEMI-
MEMBRANOSUS

QUADRICEPS,
VASTUS LATERALIS

PATELLA

HEAD OF THE FIBULA

QUADRICEPS,
VASTUS INTERMEDIUS

GASTROCNEMIUS,
LATERAL HEAD

PATELLA

FIBULA

SOLEUS

EXTENSOR
DIGITORUM LONGUS

PERONEUS
LONGUS

TIBIALIS ANTERIOR

TIBIA

PERONEUS BREVIS

CALCANEAL
TENDON

CALCANEAL
TUBEROSITY

Kneel leaning on one leg and both arms with the arms extended.

Perform a lateral leg raise (or hip abduction); maintain for a second and return to the initial position. Repeat.

This exercise engages mostly the gluteus medius and minimus, the tensor fascia lata, and, deeper, the external rotator muscle group of the hip.

This movement is performed with the leg extended or slightly flexed; it can be performed with greater amplitude in the latter part of the abduction. To work the "glute deltoid" group, combine this exercise with hip extensions on the ground during the same series.

As in all movements without extra weights, you get the best results with long series until you feel muscle burn.

Attention
Abduction of the hip is physiologically limited by the abutment of the neck of the femur against the border of the acetabulum; therefore, it is useless to try to force the leg to go higher than horizontal.

MACHINE HIP EXTENSIONS

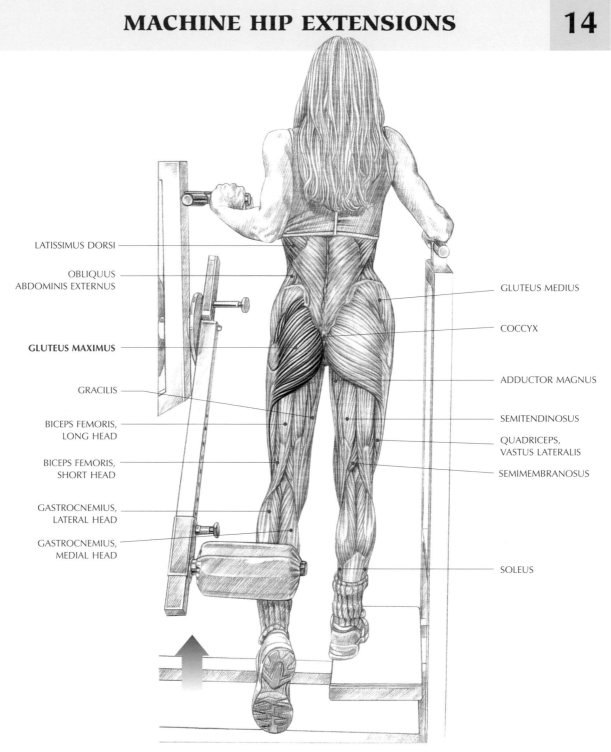

LATISSIMUS DORSI

OBLIQUUS
ABDOMINIS EXTERNUS

GLUTEUS MAXIMUS

GRACILIS

BICEPS FEMORIS,
LONG HEAD

BICEPS FEMORIS,
SHORT HEAD

GASTROCNEMIUS,
LATERAL HEAD

GASTROCNEMIUS,
MEDIAL HEAD

GLUTEUS MEDIUS

COCCYX

ADDUCTOR MAGNUS

SEMITENDINOSUS

QUADRICEPS,
VASTUS LATERALIS

SEMIMEMBRANOSUS

SOLEUS

Lean chest a bit forward, grasp handles, standing on the front leg with the pad placed at midcalf of the back leg.

Inhale and push the thigh backward to bring the hip into hyperextension. Maintain an isometric contraction for two seconds and return to beginning position. Exhale at the end of the extension.

This exercise mainly works the gluteus maximus, and to a lesser extent the semitendinosus, the semimembranosus, and the long head of the biceps femoris.

Extension of the hip at a machine allows for short series with greater weights or longer series with lesser weights.

15 STANDING HIP EXTENSIONS

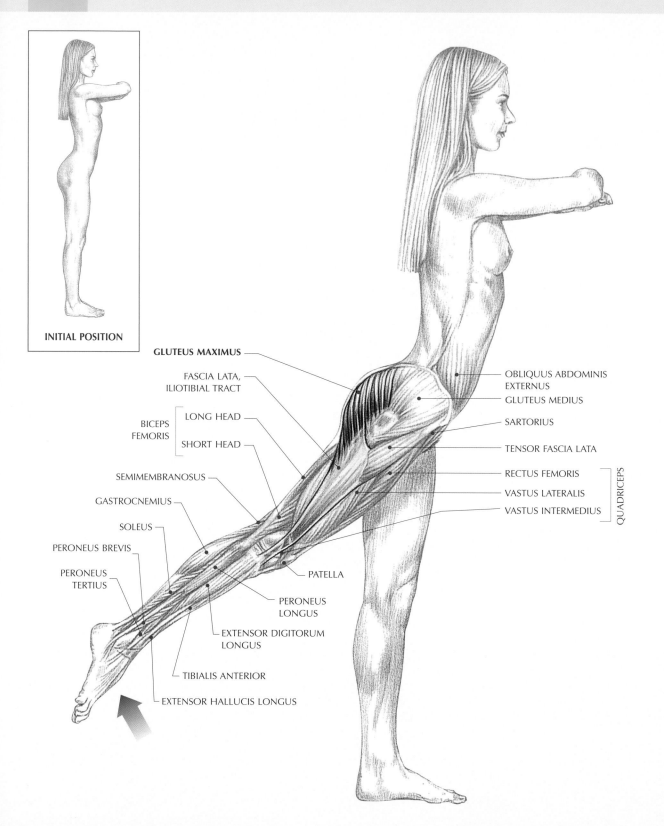

INITIAL POSITION

GLUTEUS MAXIMUS

FASCIA LATA,
ILIOTIBIAL TRACT

BICEPS
FEMORIS

LONG HEAD

SHORT HEAD

SEMIMEMBRANOSUS

GASTROCNEMIUS

SOLEUS

PERONEUS BREVIS

PERONEUS
TERTIUS

PATELLA

PERONEUS
LONGUS

EXTENSOR DIGITORUM
LONGUS

TIBIALIS ANTERIOR

EXTENSOR HALLUCIS LONGUS

OBLIQUUS ABDOMINIS
EXTERNUS

GLUTEUS MEDIUS

SARTORIUS

TENSOR FASCIA LATA

RECTUS FEMORIS

VASTUS LATERALIS

VASTUS INTERMEDIUS

QUADRICEPS

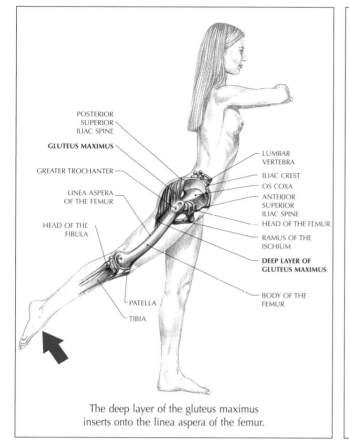

POSTERIOR
SUPERIOR
ILIAC SPINE

GLUTEUS MAXIMUS

GREATER TROCHANTER

LINEA ASPERA
OF THE FEMUR

HEAD OF THE
FIBULA

PATELLA

TIBIA

LUMBAR
VERTEBRA

ILIAC CREST

OS COXA

ANTERIOR
SUPERIOR
ILIAC SPINE

HEAD OF THE FEMUR

RAMUS OF THE
ISCHIUM

**DEEP LAYER OF
GLUTEUS MAXIMUS**

BODY OF THE
FEMUR

The deep layer of the gluteus maximus
inserts onto the linea aspera of the femur.

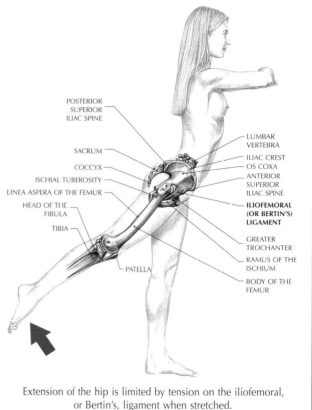

POSTERIOR
SUPERIOR
ILIAC SPINE

SACRUM

COCCYX

ISCHIAL TUBEROSITY

LINEA ASPERA OF THE FEMUR

HEAD OF THE
FIBULA

TIBIA

PATELLA

LUMBAR
VERTEBRA

ILIAC CREST

OS COXA

ANTERIOR
SUPERIOR
ILIAC SPINE

**ILIOFEMORAL
(OR BERTIN'S)
LIGAMENT**

GREATER
TROCHANTER

RAMUS OF THE
ISCHIUM

BODY OF THE
FEMUR

Extension of the hip is limited by tension on the iliofemoral,
or Bertin's, ligament when stretched.

Stand on one leg with the pelvis tilted slightly forward
and your arms crossed in front. Perform extension of the hip. Return
slowly to the initial position and repeat.

Note that extension of the hip is limited by tension on the iliofemoral,
or Bertin's, ligament when stretched.

This exercise mainly works on the gluteus maximus and to a lesser
extent the hamstring group, except for the short portion of the biceps.

As with all movements without weights, long series performed until
you feel a burn produce the best results.

For more intensity you can use ankle weights or work with an elastic
band.

For more stability the exercise can be performed while leaning on a
staff.

VARIATION WITH A STAFF

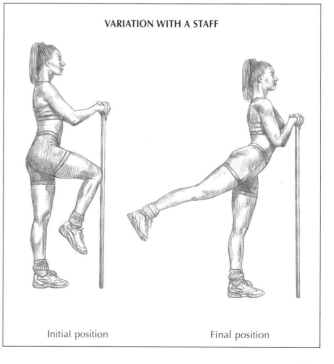

Initial position

Final position

16 FLOOR HIP EXTENSIONS

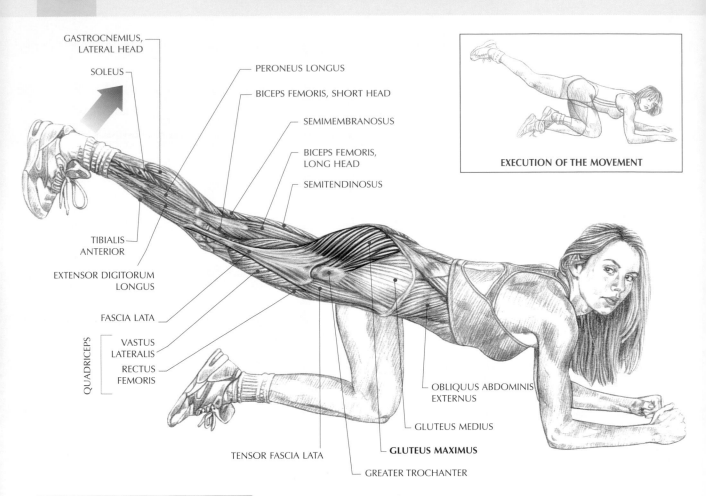

GASTROCNEMIUS, LATERAL HEAD

SOLEUS

PERONEUS LONGUS

BICEPS FEMORIS, SHORT HEAD

SEMIMEMBRANOSUS

BICEPS FEMORIS, LONG HEAD

SEMITENDINOSUS

TIBIALIS ANTERIOR

EXTENSOR DIGITORUM LONGUS

FASCIA LATA

QUADRICEPS

VASTUS LATERALIS

RECTUS FEMORIS

TENSOR FASCIA LATA

GREATER TROCHANTER

GLUTEUS MAXIMUS

GLUTEUS MEDIUS

OBLIQUUS ABDOMINIS EXTERNUS

EXECUTION OF THE MOVEMENT

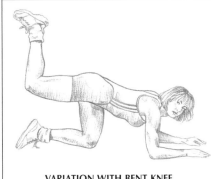

VARIATION WITH BENT KNEE

Kneel on one leg with the other one brought under the chest while resting on the forearms or the extended arms.

Bring the leg out from under the chest and backward until the hip is fully extended.

When this exercise is performed with an extended leg, it works the hamstrings and gluteus maximus; with a bent leg, only the gluteus maximus is worked but less intensely.

This movement can be performed with greater or lesser amplitude during the last part of the extension. An isometric contraction can be sustained for one or two seconds at the end of the movement. For more intensity you can use ankle weights. The ease and efficiency of this exercise have made it very popular and it is often used in group classes.

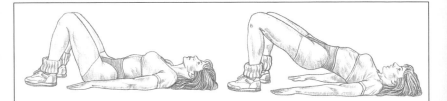

Hip raises off the floor are in fact hip extensions that mainly engage the gluteus maximus. As with the preceding movement this exercise can be performed anywhere without equipment.

MACHINE HIP EXTENSIONS
LYING DOWN

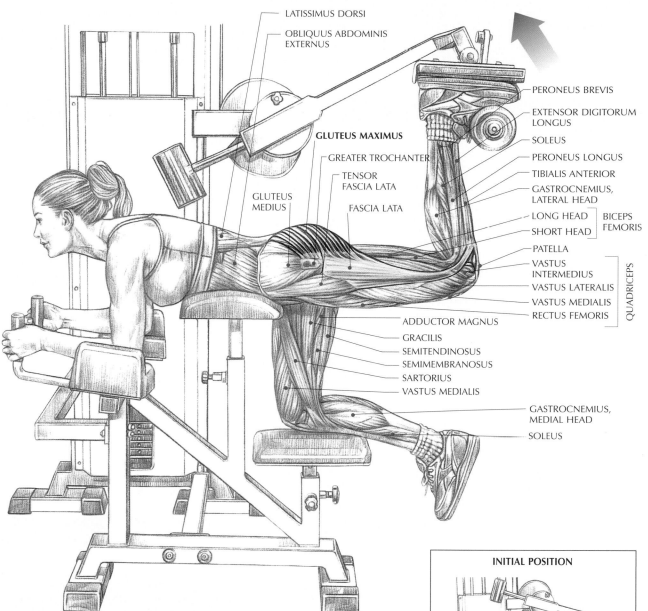

LATISSIMUS DORSI

OBLIQUUS ABDOMINIS
EXTERNUS

GLUTEUS MAXIMUS

GREATER TROCHANTER

TENSOR
FASCIA LATA

GLUTEUS
MEDIUS

FASCIA LATA

PERONEUS BREVIS

EXTENSOR DIGITORUM
LONGUS

SOLEUS

PERONEUS LONGUS

TIBIALIS ANTERIOR

GASTROCNEMIUS,
LATERAL HEAD

LONG HEAD
SHORT HEAD — BICEPS FEMORIS

PATELLA

VASTUS
INTERMEDIUS

VASTUS LATERALIS

VASTUS MEDIALIS

RECTUS FEMORIS — QUADRICEPS

ADDUCTOR MAGNUS

GRACILIS

SEMITENDINOSUS

SEMIMEMBRANOSUS

SARTORIUS

VASTUS MEDIALIS

GASTROCNEMIUS,
MEDIAL HEAD

SOLEUS

INITIAL POSITION

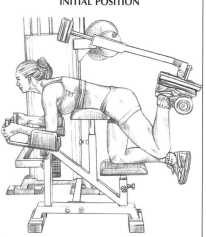

Lie prone on the apparatus, hands grasping the handles, kneeling on one leg with the other leg bent at the knee.

Inhale and push vertically with the foot on the plate until the hip is fully extended. Maintain an isometric contraction for one or two seconds, exhale and return to the initial position and repeat.

This exercise works mainly on the gluteus maximus. Note that the bent knee position relaxes the hamstrings so that these are only weakly engaged during the hip extension.

Series of 10 to 20 reps produce good results.

It is possible to work with more force by increasing the weights and reducing the number of reps.

Note

Hip extension lying down at the machine is the same movement and position as hip extension on the floor, which is popular in group classes.

18

HIP EXTENSIONS WITH A LOW PULLEY

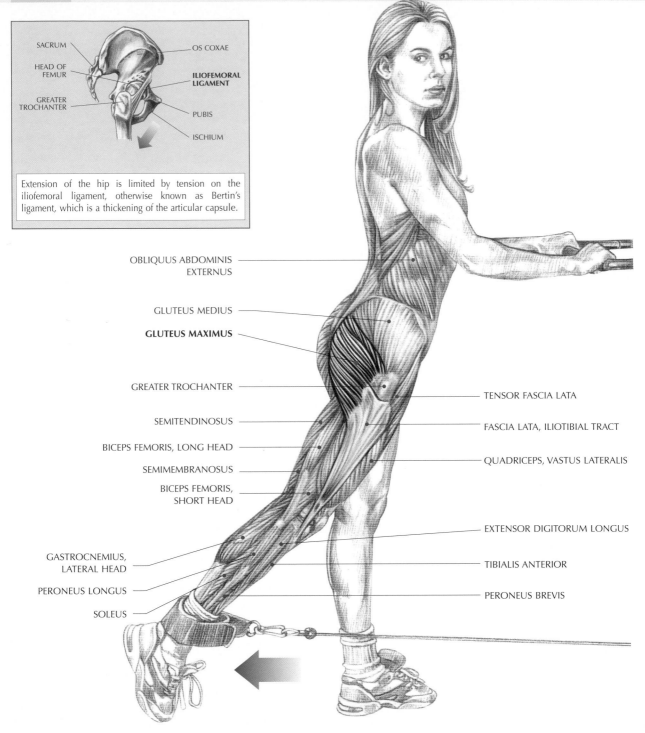

SACRUM

OS COXAE

HEAD OF FEMUR

ILIOFEMORAL LIGAMENT

GREATER TROCHANTER

PUBIS

ISCHIUM

Extension of the hip is limited by tension on the iliofemoral ligament, otherwise known as Bertin's ligament, which is a thickening of the articular capsule.

OBLIQUUS ABDOMINIS EXTERNUS

GLUTEUS MEDIUS

GLUTEUS MAXIMUS

GREATER TROCHANTER

SEMITENDINOSUS

BICEPS FEMORIS, LONG HEAD

SEMIMEMBRANOSUS

BICEPS FEMORIS, SHORT HEAD

GASTROCNEMIUS, LATERAL HEAD

PERONEUS LONGUS

SOLEUS

TENSOR FASCIA LATA

FASCIA LATA, ILIOTIBIAL TRACT

QUADRICEPS, VASTUS LATERALIS

EXTENSOR DIGITORUM LONGUS

TIBIALIS ANTERIOR

PERONEUS BREVIS

Stand on one leg facing the machine, grasping the handles, pelvis tilted forward, with the other leg connected to the low cable. Extend the hip. Note that hip extension is limited by the tension on the iliofemoral ligament (Bertin's ligament).

This exercise mainly works the gluteus maximus, and to a lesser extent the hamstrings, except for the short portion of the biceps. It helps shape as well as firm up the buttocks.

GLUTEALS, A HUMAN CHARACTERISTIC

Although certain apes occasionally practice "walking," the human is the only primate and one of the few mammals to have adopted complete biped displacement.

One of the morphological characteristics of this method of locomotion is the significant development of the gluteus maximus muscle, which has become the biggest and strongest muscle in the human body.

The development of the gluteals is truly a human characteristic, if we compare with quadrupeds, whose gluteal development is proportionately less. The horse's hindquarters, which are sometimes associated with gluteals, are in fact made up of hamstrings (the posterior part of the thigh in humans).

In the human the gluteus maximus, which is a hip extensor, does not play an important role in gait as the righting of the pelvis (that is to say, extension of the hip) is maintained by the hamstrings; one only needs to feel the gluteals while walking to notice that they are hardly contracted.

However, as soon as effort is increased—as in walking up a hill, walking fast, or running—the gluteus maximus becomes engaged to extend the hip energetically and straighten the torso.

These biomechanical ideas help us understand that when performing specific movements for the gluteus maximus and the hamstrings, as in "good mornings" (see page 72) or stiff-legged dead lifts (see page 71), the more weight we place on the gluteus maximus, the more it is solicited and the less the hamstrings are solicited.

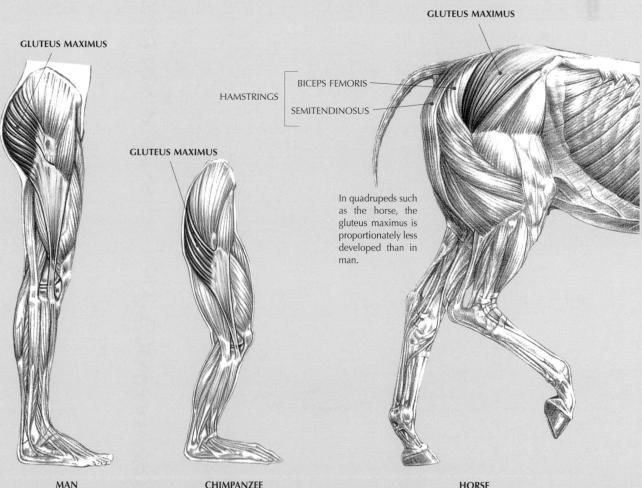

GLUTEUS MAXIMUS

GLUTEUS MAXIMUS

GLUTEUS MAXIMUS

HAMSTRINGS
BICEPS FEMORIS
SEMITENDINOSUS

In quadrupeds such as the horse, the gluteus maximus is proportionately less developed than in man.

MAN

CHIMPANZEE

HORSE

19 FLOOR HIP EXTENSIONS WITH AN ELASTIC BAND

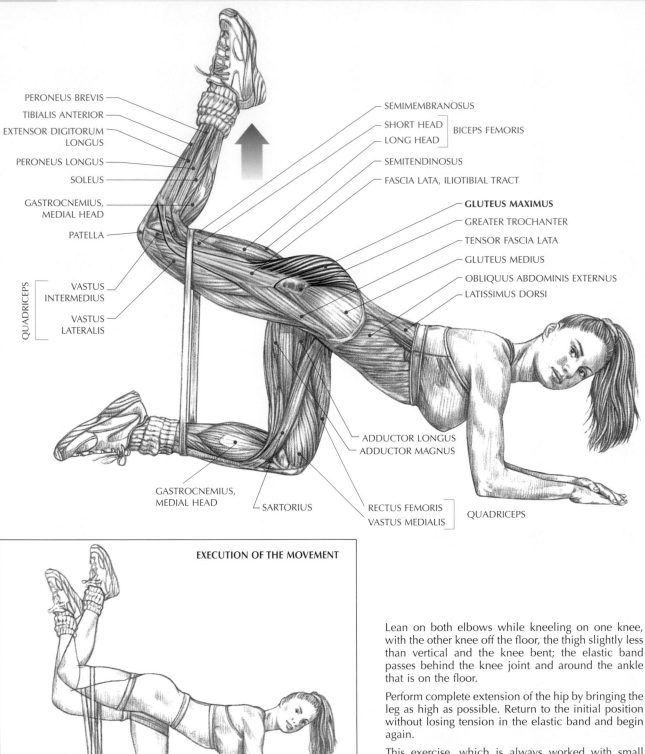

PERONEUS BREVIS
TIBIALIS ANTERIOR
EXTENSOR DIGITORUM LONGUS
PERONEUS LONGUS
SOLEUS
GASTROCNEMIUS, MEDIAL HEAD
PATELLA
QUADRICEPS
VASTUS INTERMEDIUS
VASTUS LATERALIS

SEMIMEMBRANOSUS
SHORT HEAD
LONG HEAD } BICEPS FEMORIS
SEMITENDINOSUS
FASCIA LATA, ILIOTIBIAL TRACT
GLUTEUS MAXIMUS
GREATER TROCHANTER
TENSOR FASCIA LATA
GLUTEUS MEDIUS
OBLIQUUS ABDOMINIS EXTERNUS
LATISSIMUS DORSI

ADDUCTOR LONGUS
ADDUCTOR MAGNUS

GASTROCNEMIUS, MEDIAL HEAD
SARTORIUS
RECTUS FEMORIS
VASTUS MEDIALIS } QUADRICEPS

EXECUTION OF THE MOVEMENT

Lean on both elbows while kneeling on one knee, with the other knee off the floor, the thigh slightly less than vertical and the knee bent; the elastic band passes behind the knee joint and around the ankle that is on the floor.

Perform complete extension of the hip by bringing the leg as high as possible. Return to the initial position without losing tension in the elastic band and begin again.

This exercise, which is always worked with small amplitude, works the gluteus maximus and to a lesser extent the hamstrings.

Best results occur with long series.

HIP EXTENSIONS ON A BENCH

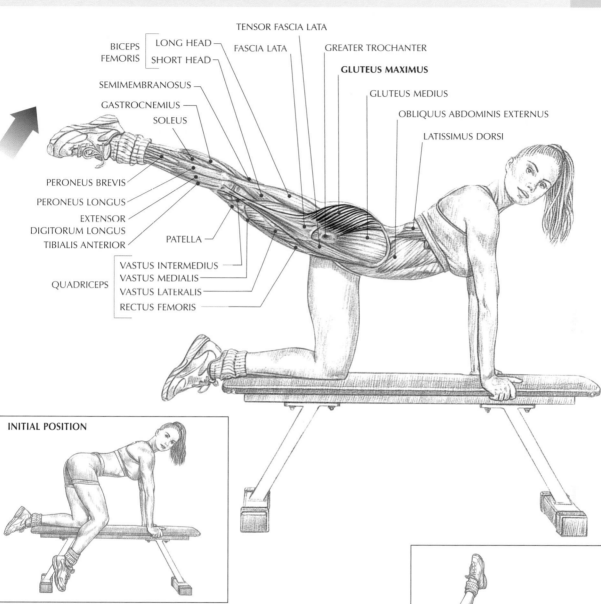

TENSOR FASCIA LATA

BICEPS FEMORIS — LONG HEAD
SHORT HEAD — FASCIA LATA

GREATER TROCHANTER

GLUTEUS MAXIMUS

GLUTEUS MEDIUS

SEMIMEMBRANOSUS

GASTROCNEMIUS

SOLEUS

OBLIQUUS ABDOMINIS EXTERNUS

LATISSIMUS DORSI

PERONEUS BREVIS

PERONEUS LONGUS

EXTENSOR DIGITORUM LONGUS

TIBIALIS ANTERIOR

PATELLA

VASTUS INTERMEDIUS
VASTUS MEDIALIS
QUADRICEPS — VASTUS LATERALIS
RECTUS FEMORIS

INITIAL POSITION

Kneel on the bench on one knee with the foot of the other leg on the floor. Lean on the hands with the arms extended, back straight or slightly arched.

Bring the leg off the floor into complete hip extension.

Return to the initial position, without touching the floor this time, and repeat.

This exercise, performed with the leg extended, works the hamstrings (biceps femoris, except for the short portion; semitendinosus; semimembranosus) as well as gluteus maximus.

While bending the knee at the end of extension at the hip you can limit the working of the hamstrings.

Unlike hip extension on the floor, this movement allows you better to feel the gluteus maximus kick in.

It is possible to maintain an isometric contraction one or two seconds at the end of extension. Ankle weights can be used to increase the intensity. Best results occur when you perform long series until you feel a burn.

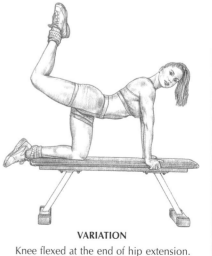

VARIATION
Knee flexed at the end of hip extension.

21 PRONE HIP EXTENSIONS

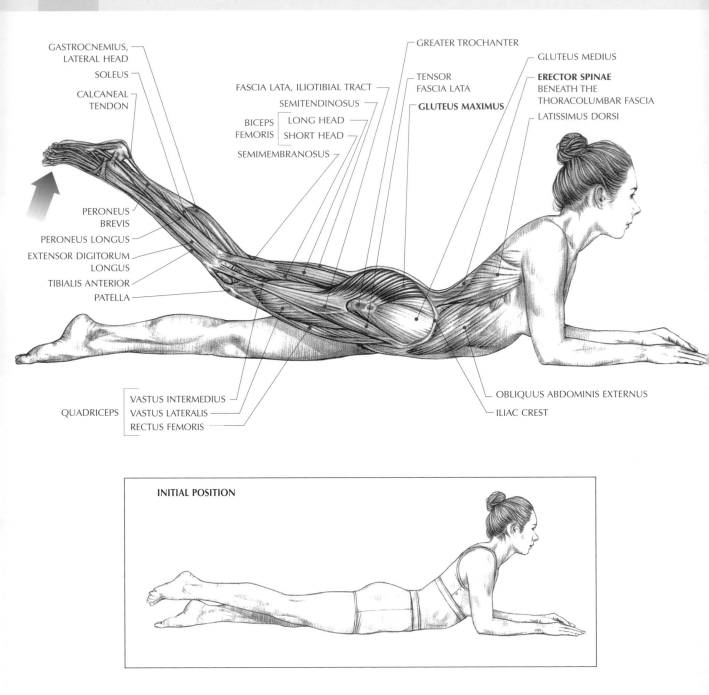

GASTROCNEMIUS,
LATERAL HEAD
SOLEUS
CALCANEAL
TENDON

PERONEUS
BREVIS
PERONEUS LONGUS
EXTENSOR DIGITORUM
LONGUS
TIBIALIS ANTERIOR
PATELLA

QUADRICEPS
VASTUS INTERMEDIUS
VASTUS LATERALIS
RECTUS FEMORIS

FASCIA LATA, ILIOTIBIAL TRACT
SEMITENDINOSUS
BICEPS
FEMORIS
LONG HEAD
SHORT HEAD
SEMIMEMBRANOSUS

GREATER TROCHANTER
TENSOR
FASCIA LATA
GLUTEUS MAXIMUS

GLUTEUS MEDIUS
ERECTOR SPINAE
BENEATH THE
THORACOLUMBAR FASCIA
LATISSIMUS DORSI

OBLIQUUS ABDOMINIS EXTERNUS
ILIAC CREST

INITIAL POSITION

Lie prone on your stomach, leaning on your forearms with the upper arms vertical and the back slightly arched, one leg raised slightly off the floor. Raise the raised leg as high as possible and return to the initial position without touching the floor with that foot. Repeat.

This exercise, worked in long series, works mainly the gluteus maximus and to a lesser degree the hamstrings and the lumbosacral erector spinae muscle group, located in the lower back.

Variation
Between each repetition you may hold the leg raised for one or two seconds in an isometric contraction.

STANDING HIP EXTENSIONS
WITH AN ELASTIC BAND

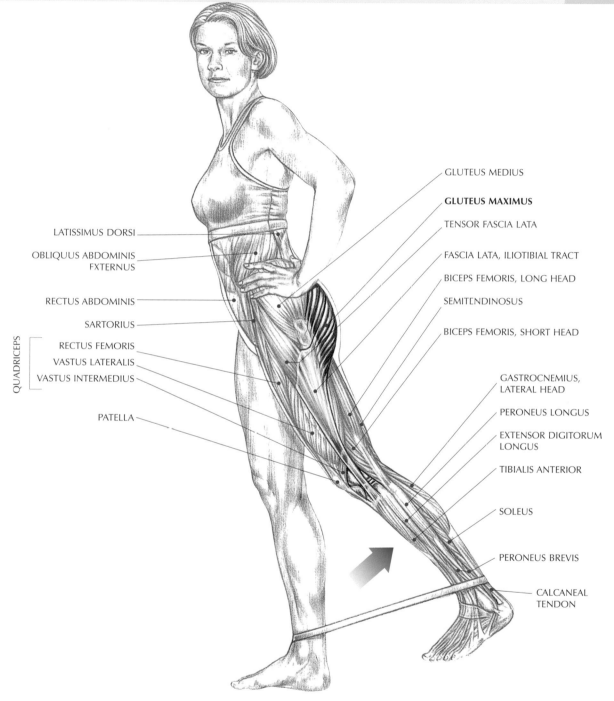

GLUTEUS MEDIUS

GLUTEUS MAXIMUS

TENSOR FASCIA LATA

FASCIA LATA, ILIOTIBIAL TRACT

BICEPS FEMORIS, LONG HEAD

SEMITENDINOSUS

BICEPS FEMORIS, SHORT HEAD

GASTROCNEMIUS, LATERAL HEAD

PERONEUS LONGUS

EXTENSOR DIGITORUM LONGUS

TIBIALIS ANTERIOR

SOLEUS

PERONEUS BREVIS

CALCANEAL TENDON

LATISSIMUS DORSI

OBLIQUUS ABDOMINIS EXTERNUS

RECTUS ABDOMINIS

SARTORIUS

QUADRICEPS
RECTUS FEMORIS
VASTUS LATERALIS
VASTUS INTERMEDIUS

PATELLA

Stand on one leg with your hands on your hips and the elastic band stretched around both ankles.

Extend the hip and return to the initial position, maintaining the tension of the elastic band. Begin again.

As with all movements performed with an elastic band, best results occur with long series until you feel a burn.

This exercise works mainly on the gluteus maximus and to a lesser extent the hamstring group, with the exception of the short head of biceps femoris, which only flexes the leg and therefore does not participate in extension of the hip.

23 PELVIC RAISES OFF THE FLOOR

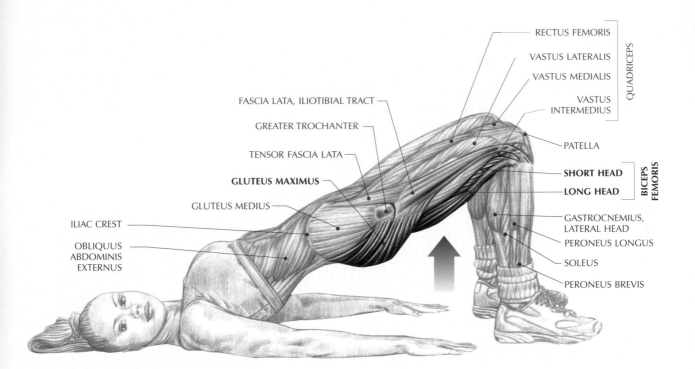

RECTUS FEMORIS
VASTUS LATERALIS
VASTUS MEDIALIS
VASTUS INTERMEDIUS
QUADRICEPS

FASCIA LATA, ILIOTIBIAL TRACT
GREATER TROCHANTER
TENSOR FASCIA LATA
GLUTEUS MAXIMUS
GLUTEUS MEDIUS
ILIAC CREST
OBLIQUUS ABDOMINIS EXTERNUS

PATELLA
SHORT HEAD
LONG HEAD
BICEPS FEMORIS
GASTROCNEMIUS, LATERAL HEAD
PERONEUS LONGUS
SOLEUS
PERONEUS BREVIS

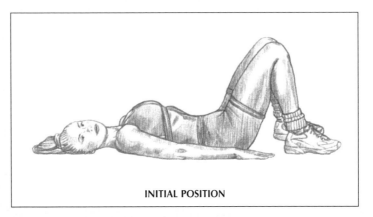

INITIAL POSITION

Lie on your back with arms along your sides, palms down, and knees flexed.

Inhale, push down through the feet, and lift the buttocks off the floor. Hold the position for two seconds and lower the pelvis without touching the floor with the buttocks.

Exhale and start again.

This exercise mainly works the hamstrings and gluteus maximus.

It is performed in long series, and it is important to feel the muscle contraction at the end of the hip raise.

Note

This hip raise off the floor is easy and effective and has become part of most group classes.

PELVIC RAISES ON ONE LEG

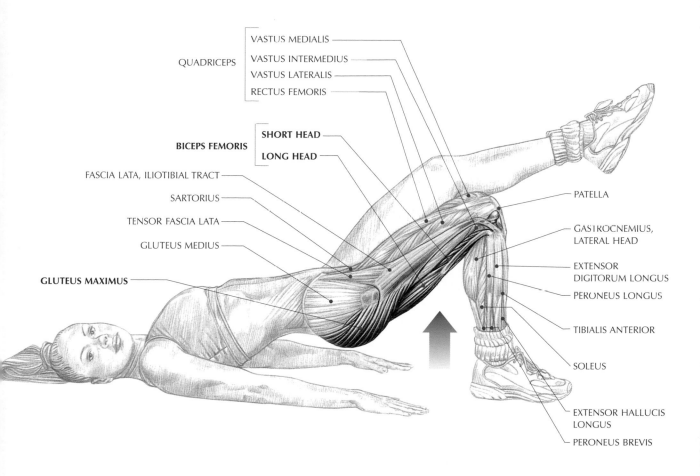

QUADRICEPS
- VASTUS MEDIALIS
- VASTUS INTERMEDIUS
- VASTUS LATERALIS
- RECTUS FEMORIS

BICEPS FEMORIS
- **SHORT HEAD**
- **LONG HEAD**

FASCIA LATA, ILIOTIBIAL TRACT

SARTORIUS

TENSOR FASCIA LATA

GLUTEUS MEDIUS

GLUTEUS MAXIMUS

PATELLA

GASTROCNEMIUS, LATERAL HEAD

EXTENSOR DIGITORUM LONGUS

PERONEUS LONGUS

TIBIALIS ANTERIOR

SOLEUS

EXTENSOR HALLUCIS LONGUS

PERONEUS BREVIS

Lie on your back with arms alongside the body, palms down, one leg bent on the floor, the other leg extended forward and not touching the floor.

Inhale and raise the buttocks, pushing as hard as possible through the foot on the floor.

Maintain the position two seconds and lower the pelvis without touching the floor. Exhale and begin again.

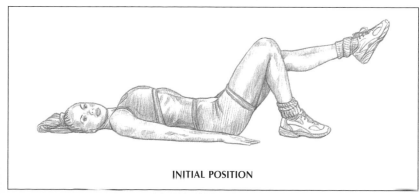

INITIAL POSITION

This exercise mainly works the hamstrings (semitendinosus, semimembranosus, biceps femoris) and the gluteus maximus.

It is performed in long series; the important thing is to feel the muscle contractions at the end of the hip raise.

Note

Complete series may be performed on one side and then the other, or by alternating sides during the same series from right leg to left leg, resting the back on the floor between each repetition.

25   PELVIC RAISES OFF A BENCH

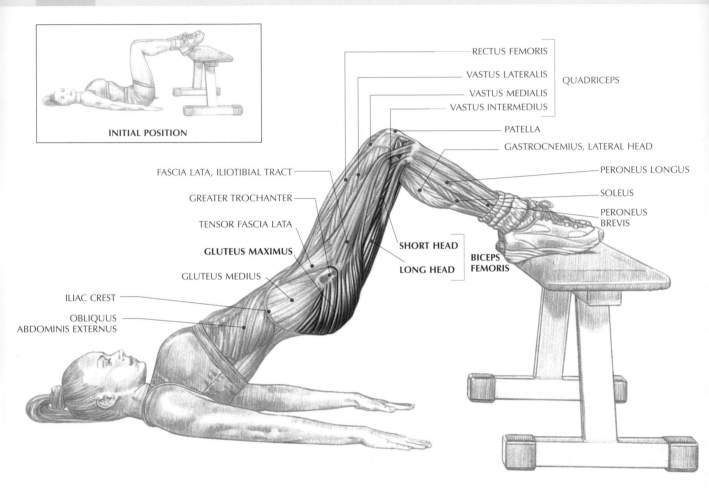

INITIAL POSITION

RECTUS FEMORIS

VASTUS LATERALIS

QUADRICEPS

VASTUS MEDIALIS

VASTUS INTERMEDIUS

PATELLA

GASTROCNEMIUS, LATERAL HEAD

PERONEUS LONGUS

SOLEUS

PERONEUS BREVIS

FASCIA LATA, ILIOTIBIAL TRACT

GREATER TROCHANTER

TENSOR FASCIA LATA

GLUTEUS MAXIMUS

GLUTEUS MEDIUS

ILIAC CREST

OBLIQUUS ABDOMINIS EXTERNUS

SHORT HEAD

LONG HEAD

BICEPS FEMORIS

Lie on your back, arms alongside the body, palms down, thighs vertical, and feet resting on a bench.

Inhale and raise the hips off the floor; maintain the position two seconds and lower without touching the floor.

Exhale and begin again.

This exercise works the gluteus maximus and especially the hamstrings; this latter group is worked far more than with the pelvic raise off the floor (see page 38).

This movement is executed slowly; the important thing is to feel the muscle contraction.

Series of 10 to 15 repetitions give the best results.

Note

It is important to note that pelvic raises are in fact extensions of the hip.

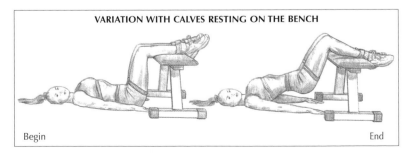

VARIATION WITH CALVES RESTING ON THE BENCH

Begin

End

Variations

- It is possible to perform the movement with small amplitude without lowering the pelvis down to the floor too much, feeling for the muscle burn.
- When you raise the pelvis with the calves resting on the bench, the hamstrings are more intensely worked with associated intense work of the gastrocnemii.

POSTERIOR PELVIC TILTS

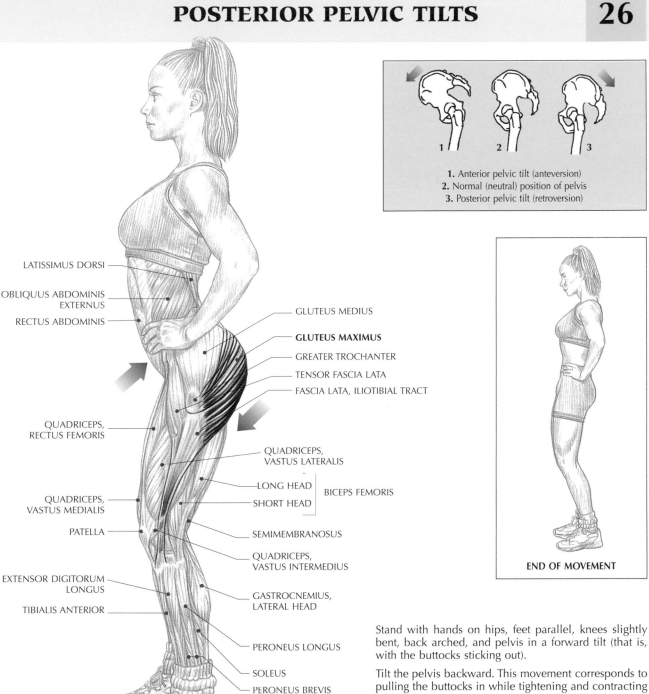

1. Anterior pelvic tilt (anteversion)
2. Normal (neutral) position of pelvis
3. Posterior pelvic tilt (retroversion)

LATISSIMUS DORSI

OBLIQUUS ABDOMINIS EXTERNUS

RECTUS ABDOMINIS

GLUTEUS MEDIUS

GLUTEUS MAXIMUS

GREATER TROCHANTER

TENSOR FASCIA LATA

FASCIA LATA, ILIOTIBIAL TRACT

QUADRICEPS, RECTUS FEMORIS

QUADRICEPS, VASTUS LATERALIS

LONG HEAD

SHORT HEAD

BICEPS FEMORIS

QUADRICEPS, VASTUS MEDIALIS

PATELLA

SEMIMEMBRANOSUS

QUADRICEPS, VASTUS INTERMEDIUS

EXTENSOR DIGITORUM LONGUS

TIBIALIS ANTERIOR

GASTROCNEMIUS, LATERAL HEAD

PERONEUS LONGUS

SOLEUS

PERONEUS BREVIS

END OF MOVEMENT

Stand with hands on hips, feet parallel, knees slightly bent, back arched, and pelvis in a forward tilt (that is, with the buttocks sticking out).

Tilt the pelvis backward. This movement corresponds to pulling the buttocks in while tightening and contracting to the max for two or three seconds. Return to the initial position and begin again.

This exercise mainly works the gluteus maximus and deeper in, the external rotators of the hip (piriformis, obturator internus, superior and inferior gemelli—all except the obturator externus).

Not as effective as exercises with weights, posterior pelvic tilts only work in long series.

This is an excellent beginner movement that helps to develop awareness of the function of the gluteus maximus.

For best results, combine this movement in your workout with an exercise with weights

27 SMALL LATERAL THIGH FLEXIONS

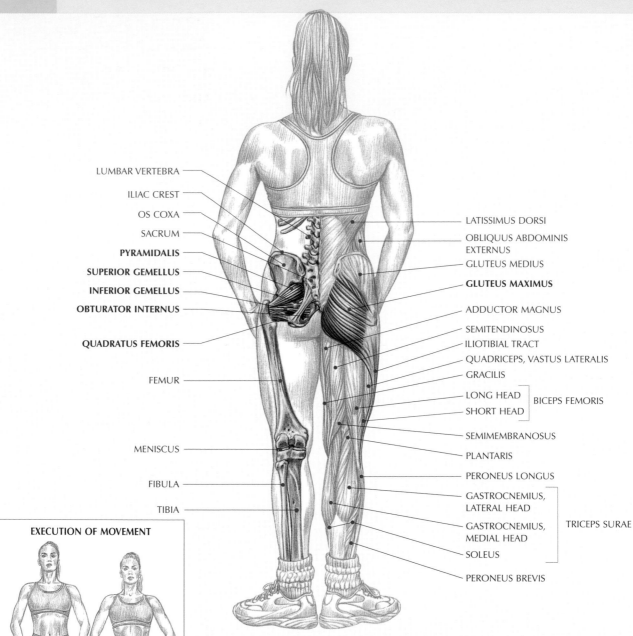

LUMBAR VERTEBRA

ILIAC CREST

OS COXA

SACRUM

PYRAMIDALIS

SUPERIOR GEMELLUS

INFERIOR GEMELLUS

OBTURATOR INTERNUS

QUADRATUS FEMORIS

FEMUR

MENISCUS

FIBULA

TIBIA

LATISSIMUS DORSI

OBLIQUUS ABDOMINIS EXTERNUS

GLUTEUS MEDIUS

GLUTEUS MAXIMUS

ADDUCTOR MAGNUS

SEMITENDINOSUS

ILIOTIBIAL TRACT

QUADRICEPS, VASTUS LATERALIS

GRACILIS

LONG HEAD
SHORT HEAD } BICEPS FEMORIS

SEMIMEMBRANOSUS

PLANTARIS

PERONEUS LONGUS

GASTROCNEMIUS, LATERAL HEAD

GASTROCNEMIUS, MEDIAL HEAD } TRICEPS SURAE

SOLEUS

PERONEUS BREVIS

EXECUTION OF MOVEMENT

1. Initial position
2. Bent thighs

Stand with hands on thighs, back straight and toes turned out, heels touching, with the feet in the axis of the knees. (Be careful: the amount of turn-out and flexibility at the hips varies from person to person, so that it is useless to turn the feet out completely if you do not have that flexibility.)

Bend the knees about a third of the way down and return to the initial position by squeezing the glutes to the max for three or four seconds.

The muscles that are mainly engaged are the gluteus maximus and, deeper in, the external rotators of the thigh (pyramidalis, quadratus femoris, obturator internus, and superior and inferior gemelli of the hip).

Perform this exercise slowly while focusing on the feel of the muscles. As with most movements that use the body weight, results only occur in long series.

To feel the working of the gluteus maximus at the end of the series, maintain an isometric contraction by strongly squeezing the glutes for 20 seconds more or less.

LEGS

II

1. SQUATS

2. SQUATS WITH A STAFF

3. SQUATS WITH LEGS APART

4. SQUATS WITH A BAR IN FRONT

5. SQUATS WITH AN ELASTIC BAND

6. ANTERIOR SQUATS WITH A STAFF

7. SQUATS AT A FRAME GUIDE

8. THIGH FLEXIONS
   IN A ROMAN CHAIR

9. THIGH FLEXIONS WITH DUMBBELLS

10. THIGH FLEXIONS

11. THIGH FLEXIONS WITH LEGS APART

12. ALTERNATING LATERAL LUNGES

13. FLEXIONS ON ONE LEG

14. HACK SQUATS

15. THIGHS AT AN INCLINE PRESS

16. LEG EXTENSIONS AT AN INCLINE MACHINE

17. THIGH RAISES

18. THIGH RAISES WITH WEIGHTS

19. ADDUCTORS ON THE FLOOR

20. ADDUCTORS AT A LOW PULLEY

21. ADDUCTORS AT A MACHINE

22. ADDUCTORS WITH A BALL

23. STIFF-LEGGED DEAD LIFTS

24. GOOD MORNINGS

25. GOOD MORNINGS WITH A STAFF

26. LYING LEG CURLS

27. STANDING LEG CURLS

28. SEATED LEG CURLS

29. HAMSTRINGS AT A BENCH

30. HAMSTRINGS ON THE FLOOR

31. KNEELING HAMSTRINGS

32. STANDING CALF RAISES

33. DONKEY CALF RAISES

34. ONE-LEG TOE RAISES

35. STANDING BARBELL CALF RAISES

36. SEATED BARBELL CALF RAISES

37. SEATED CALF RAISES

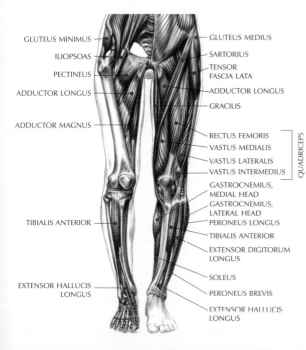

GLUTEUS MINIMUS
ILIOPSOAS
PECTINEUS
ADDUCTOR LONGUS
ADDUCTOR MAGNUS
TIBIALIS ANTERIOR
EXTENSOR HALLUCIS LONGUS

GLUTEUS MEDIUS
SARTORIUS
TENSOR FASCIA LATA
ADDUCTOR LONGUS
GRACILIS
RECTUS FEMORIS
VASTUS MEDIALIS
VASTUS LATERALIS
VASTUS INTERMEDIUS
QUADRICEPS
GASTROCNEMIUS, MEDIAL HEAD
GASTROCNEMIUS, LATERAL HEAD
PERONEUS LONGUS
TIBIALIS ANTERIOR
EXTENSOR DIGITORUM LONGUS
SOLEUS
PERONEUS BREVIS
EXTENSOR HALLUCIS LONGUS

GLUTEUS MINIMUS
PIRIFORMIS
SUPERIOR GEMELLUS
OBTURATOR INTERNUS
INFERIOR GEMELLUS
QUADRATUS FEMORIS
BICEPS FEMORIS, LONG HEAD
SEMITENDINOSUS
BICEPS FEMORIS, SHORT HEAD
SEMIMEMBRANOSUS
POPLITEUS
PERONEUS LONGUS
FLEXOR DIGITORUM LONGUS
TIBIALIS POSTERIOR
FLEXOR HALLUCIS LONGUS
PERONEUS BREVIS

GLUTEUS MEDIUS
GLUTEUS MAXIMUS
GREATER TROCHANTER
TENSOR FASCIA LATA
ADDUCTOR MAGNUS
FASCIA LATA, ILIOTIBIAL TRACT
GRACILIS
SEMITENDINOSUS
BICEPS FEMORIS, LONG HEAD
SEMIMEMBRANOSUS
BICEPS FEMORIS, SHORT HEAD
SARTORIUS
PLANTARIS
GASTROCNEMIUS, LATERAL HEAD
GASTROCNEMIUS, MEDIAL HEAD
SOLEUS
PERONEUS LONGUS
PERONEUS BREVIS

MORPHOLOGICAL DIFFERENCES BETWEEN WOMEN AND MEN

The morphological differences between women and men are the result of differences in the volume and proportion of similar anatomical features. Generally speaking, the female skeleton is not as massive; it is smoother and more delicate with impressions—hollows or bumps—that serve as muscle insertions or provide passage for tendons, which are less accentuated. (The more highly developed musculature in men marks the skeleton more.) The female thoracic cage is generally more rounded and not as big as in the male. Proportionately, the skeletal width of the shoulders is the same as in the male, but the larger muscular development of the latter makes it seem wider. The lumbar curve is greater in women and the pelvis is tilted anteriorly (anteversion), which makes for the sway-backed appearance often found in women. If the waist in women is longer and smaller, it is because the thorax is more constricted at the base and the pelvis is generally not as high.

The most important difference between the male and female skeletons is found at the level of the pelvis. The female pelvis is adapted for gestation: it is not as high and is proportionately wider than that of the male. The sacrum of the female is wider and the pelvic ring is wider and more circular to facilitate the passage of the newborn. As the pelvic ring is wider, the acetabula (the fossa in which the heads of the femurs lodge) are farther apart, which increases the distance between the greater trochanters and consequently the width of the hips.

COMPARISON BETWEEN THE MALE AND FEMALE PELVIS SHOWING THE INFLUENCE OF THE SKELETON ON THE EXTERNAL SHAPE

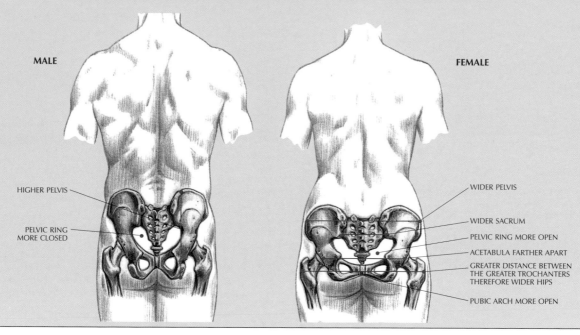

MALE

HIGHER PELVIS

PELVIC RING MORE CLOSED

FEMALE

WIDER PELVIS

WIDER SACRUM

PELVIC RING MORE OPEN

ACETABULA FARTHER APART

GREATER DISTANCE BETWEEN THE GREATER TROCHANTERS THEREFORE WIDER HIPS

PUBIC ARCH MORE OPEN

COMPARISON BETWEEN THE INFERIOR PELVIC OPENINGS IN THE MALE AND FEMALE

*Notice that the pelvic ring is wider and more circular in women.

Wider and more open than the male pelvis, the female pelvis is built for childbirth

COCCYX SACRUM SACROTUBEROUS LIGAMENT

ALA OF THE ILIUM

ISCHIAL TUBEROSITY

RAMUS OF THE ISCHIUM

PUBIC SYMPHYSIS PUBIS

ACETABULUM

MALE PELVIS

FEMALE PELVIS

DIAGRAM OF A FEMALE PELVIS SHOWING THE CRANIUM OF A NEONATE

Greater hip width in women influences the position of the femurs, which are often more angled than in men, giving them a slight X shape.

A wide pelvis with a significant angle of the femur can provoke genu valgum, accentuated all the more by the hyperlaxity toward which women tend. The legs then take on a typical X shape: the articulation at the knee is excessively solicited; the medial collateral ligament is overstretched; and the lateral meniscus, the cartilage-covered articular surfaces of the external condyle of the femur, and the lateral tuberosity of the tibia are subjected to excessive loads, which may lead to premature wear.

Pathological genu valgum is accompanied by medial collapse at the ankle and the disappearance of the plantar arch (flat foot), which may involve pain because of excessive stretching of certain muscles in the sole of the foot.

It is very important to take into account the individual morphologies and to remember that women are more often prone to genu valgum pathologies, whereas men more frequently suffer from bow-legs (genu varum). People with very noticeable genu valgum should therefore work out carefully, avoid training with heavy weights, and always perform the movements so as to avoid impacts that would aggravate knee and ankle problems.

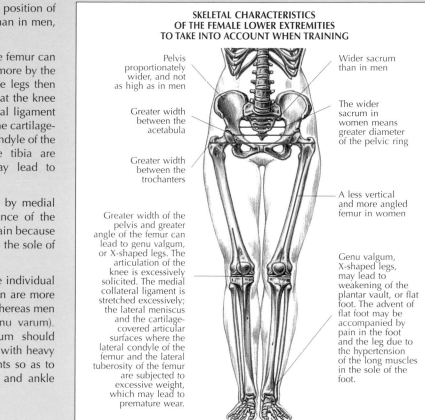

SKELETAL CHARACTERISTICS OF THE FEMALE LOWER EXTREMITIES TO TAKE INTO ACCOUNT WHEN TRAINING

Pelvis proportionately wider, and not as high as in men

Greater width between the acetabula

Greater width between the trochanters

Greater width of the pelvis and greater angle of the femur can lead to genu valgum, or X-shaped legs. The articulation of the knee is excessively solicited. The medial collateral ligament is stretched excessively; the lateral meniscus and the cartilage-covered articular surfaces where the lateral condyle of the femur and the lateral tuberosity of the femur are subjected to excessive weight, which may lead to premature wear.

Wider sacrum than in men

The wider sacrum in women means greater diameter of the pelvic ring

A less vertical and more angled femur in women

Genu valgum, X-shaped legs, may lead to weakening of the plantar vault, or flat foot. The advent of flat foot may be accompanied by pain in the foot and the leg due to the hypertension of the long muscles in the sole of the foot.

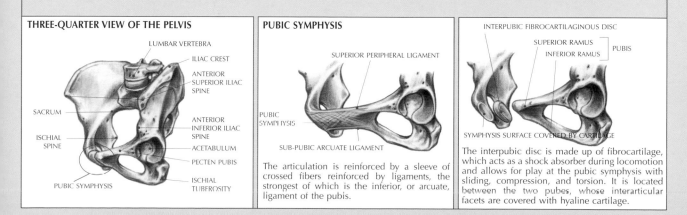

DISLOCATION OF THE PUBIC SYMPHYSIS

The increased secretion of certain hormones during pregnancy, especially relaxin, induces muscle relaxation and even greater ligament suppleness. This temporary ligamentous hyperlaxity is especially important at the level of the articulations in the pelvis, which are generally not that mobile.

During labor, the interlocking mechanisms are not as effective, and the pubic symphysis distends, which relaxes the pelvic ring to increase the diameter and facilitate the passage of the baby. Therefore it is important after labor and birth to begin training again carefully, allowing time for the ligaments to return to their initial elasticity and avoiding movements with heavy weights, such as squats or lifts from the ground, and high impact movements on the ground, such as bench steps or step work. A return to training too soon or too hard could lead to dislocation of the pubic symphysis by ligament distension. The articulation then becomes too mobile or painful. It is particularly incapacitating for walking. Dislocation of the pubic symphysis can also occur during labor.

THREE-QUARTER VIEW OF THE PELVIS

LUMBAR VERTEBRA
ILIAC CREST
ANTERIOR SUPERIOR ILIAC SPINE
SACRUM
ANTERIOR INFERIOR ILIAC SPINE
ISCHIAL SPINE
ACETABULUM
PECTEN PUBIS
PUBIC SYMPHYSIS
ISCHIAL TUBEROSITY

PUBIC SYMPHYSIS

SUPERIOR PERIPHERAL LIGAMENT
PUBIC SYMPHYSIS
SUB-PUBIC ARCUATE LIGAMENT

The articulation is reinforced by a sleeve of crossed fibers reinforced by ligaments, the strongest of which is the inferior, or arcuate, ligament of the pubis.

INTERPUBIC FIBROCARTILAGINOUS DISC
SUPERIOR RAMUS
INFERIOR RAMUS
PUBIS
SYMPHYSIS SURFACE COVERED BY CARTILAGE

The interpubic disc is made up of fibrocartilage, which acts as a shock absorber during locomotion and allows for play at the pubic symphysis with sliding, compression, and torsion. It is located between the two pubes, whose interarticular facets are covered with hyaline cartilage.

SQUATS

1

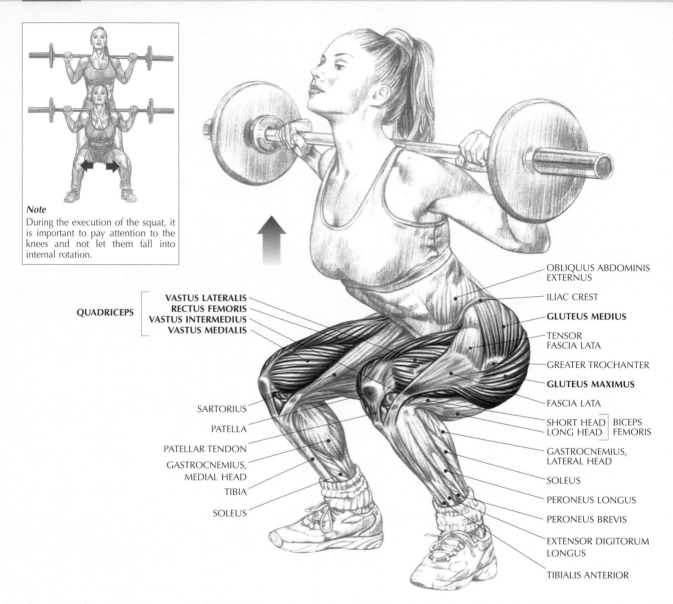

Note

During the execution of the squat, it is important to pay attention to the knees and not let them fall into internal rotation.

QUADRICEPS
- VASTUS LATERALIS
- RECTUS FEMORIS
- VASTUS INTERMEDIUS
- VASTUS MEDIALIS

SARTORIUS

PATELLA

PATELLAR TENDON

GASTROCNEMIUS, MEDIAL HEAD

TIBIA

SOLEUS

OBLIQUUS ABDOMINIS EXTERNUS

ILIAC CREST

GLUTEUS MEDIUS

TENSOR FASCIA LATA

GREATER TROCHANTER

GLUTEUS MAXIMUS

FASCIA LATA

SHORT HEAD | BICEPS
LONG HEAD | FEMORIS

GASTROCNEMIUS, LATERAL HEAD

SOLEUS

PERONEUS LONGUS

PERONEUS BREVIS

EXTENSOR DIGITORUM LONGUS

TIBIALIS ANTERIOR

The squat is the premiere movement of weightlifting, as it engages most of the muscle system; it is also excellent for the cardiovascular system. It helps achieve good thoracic expansion, which by the same token means good respiratory capacity.

With the barbell resting in a stand, slide underneath and place the barbell on the trapezius a little higher than the posterior deltoids. Grasp the bar fully in both hands (the width between the hands varies according to morphologies) and pull the elbows backward.

Take in a deep breath (to maintain an intrathoracic breath, which will prevent the chest from collapsing anteriorly). Arch the back slightly with a slight anterior pelvic tilt, contract the abdominal muscles, look straight ahead, and remove the bar from its support. Step back one or two steps and stop with the feet parallel (or with the toes slightly out), more or less shoulder width apart. Squat by leaning forward with the back (the axis of flexion passes through the coxofemoral joint) and control the descent without ever rounding the back, to avoid trauma. When the femurs are horizontal, extend the legs by raising the chest until in the beginning position. Breathe out at the end of the movement.

The squat works mainly on the quadriceps, the gluteals, the adductor mass, the erector muscles of the spine, and the abdominals, as well as the hamstrings.

THE TWO WAYS OF HOLDING THE BAR

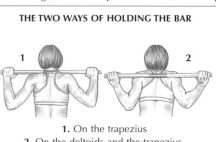

1. On the trapezius
2. On the deltoids and the trapezius, in the powerlift style

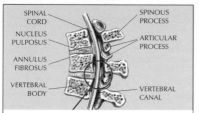

SPINAL CORD
NUCLEUS PULPOSUS
ANNULUS FIBROSUS
VERTEBRAL BODY
SPINOUS PROCESS
ARTICULAR PROCESS
VERTEBRAL CANAL

During vertebral flexion the disc is pinched anteriorly, the vertebra gaps posteriorly, and the liquid of the nucleus pulposus migrates posteriorly and can compress against the neural components (as occurs in sciatica).

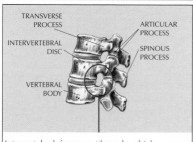

TRANSVERSE PROCESS
INTERVERTEBRAL DISC
VERTEBRAL BODY
ARTICULAR PROCESS
SPINOUS PROCESS

Intervertebral foramen (through which a nerve from the spinal cord passes)

Note

The squat is the best movement for developing the curve (shape) of the buttocks.

Variations

- For people with stiff ankles or long femurs, a block may be placed under the heels to avoid too much tilting of the torso. This variation places some of the effort onto the quadriceps.

- By varying the position of the bar on the back—that is to say, by lowering it onto the posterior deltoids—the cantilever is reduced, increasing the power of the leverage of the back, which allows for heavier weights. This technique is the one essentially used by powerlifters.

- The squat may be performed at a frame guide, which helps avoid the tilt of the torso and focuses on the quadriceps.

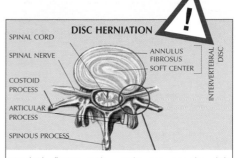

DISC HERNIATION

SPINAL CORD
SPINAL NERVE
COSTOID PROCESS
ARTICULAR PROCESS
SPINOUS PROCESS
ANNULUS FIBROSUS
SOFT CENTER
INTERVERTEBRAL DISC

Vertebral flexion with weight can provoke disk herniation, generally located at the level of the lumbar vertebrae. These herniations are frequent with squats and dead lifts and are most often the result of a poor position following a lack of proper technique.

HOW TO PLACE THE FEET IN A SQUAT

When performing a classic squat, with the feet about shoulder width apart, it is important to take into account the direction of the feet. These should be more or less parallel or with the toes pointing slightly outward. In any case the individual morphology must be respected and the feet placed in line with the knees.

Example: if you walk with the feet in a "duck waddle" perform your squat with "duck waddle" feet.

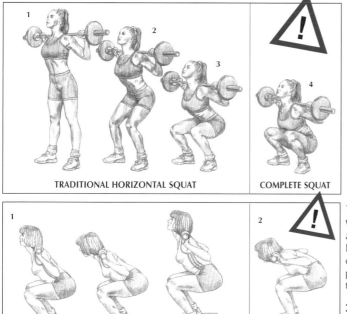

TRADITIONAL HORIZONTAL SQUAT   COMPLETE SQUAT

1-2-3 : negative phase
To feel the gluteal muscles working, it is important to bring the thighs to horizontal.

4. To better feel the working of the buttocks, the thighs can be lowered below horizontal, but this technique can only be performed by people with very supple ankles or with short femurs. Furthermore, the squat has to be performed carefully as it tends to round the back, which can lead to serious injury.

1. GOOD POSITIONS

When you are performing squats, the back should always be as straight as possible. Depending on the different morphologies (more or less long legs, or more or less stiff ankles) and different performance (width of the feet, use of compensating soles or lifts, bar in high or low position), the torso may be more or less inclined as flexion occurs at the coxofemoral level.

2. POOR POSITION

Never round the back when performing squats. This fault is responsible for most lumbar spine injuries and especially herniated discs.

Whatever the movement, as soon as it is being performed with a heavy weight it is important to "block":

- Taking a deep breath to fill the chest and holding it fills the lungs like a balloon, which makes the rib cage rigid and prevents the torso from tilting forward.
- Contracting the abdominal muscle group solidifies the stomach and increases intra-abdominal pressure, which prevents the torso from tilting forward.
- Finally, contracting the lumbar muscles to arch the low back puts the spinal column into extension.

These three actions performed simultaneously are called **"blocking"** and prevent rounding the back, or vertebral flexion, a position that, with heavy weights, predisposes to the all-too-familiar disc herniation.

2 SQUATS WITH A STAFF

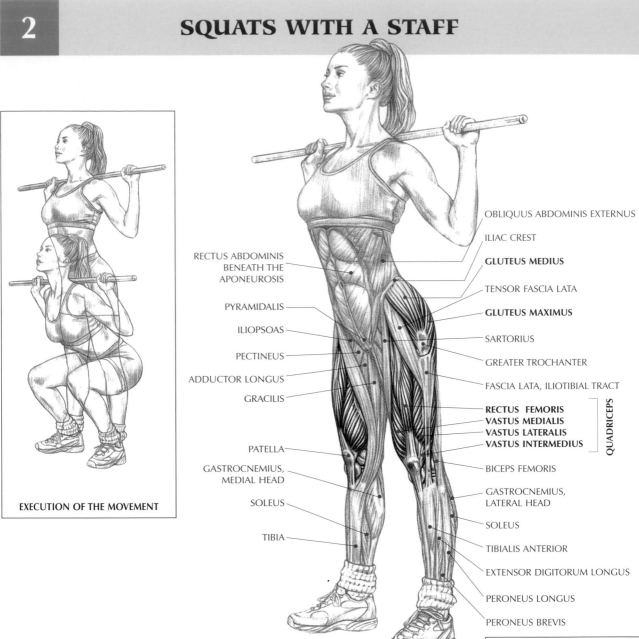

OBLIQUUS ABDOMINIS EXTERNUS

ILIAC CREST

GLUTEUS MEDIUS

TENSOR FASCIA LATA

GLUTEUS MAXIMUS

SARTORIUS

GREATER TROCHANTER

FASCIA LATA, ILIOTIBIAL TRACT

RECTUS FEMORIS
VASTUS MEDIALIS
VASTUS LATERALIS
VASTUS INTERMEDIUS

QUADRICEPS

BICEPS FEMORIS

GASTROCNEMIUS, LATERAL HEAD

SOLEUS

TIBIALIS ANTERIOR

EXTENSOR DIGITORUM LONGUS

PERONEUS LONGUS

PERONEUS BREVIS

RECTUS ABDOMINIS BENEATH THE APONEUROSIS

PYRAMIDALIS

ILIOPSOAS

PECTINEUS

ADDUCTOR LONGUS

GRACILIS

PATELLA

GASTROCNEMIUS, MEDIAL HEAD

SOLEUS

TIBIA

EXECUTION OF THE MOVEMENT

Stand with the feet more or less shoulder width apart, the chest out, and the back slightly arched, the staff resting on the trapezius a little above the posterior deltoids.

Inhale, contract the abdominal muscles, and crouch without ever rounding the back or lifting the heels off the floor. When the thighs are horizontal, extend the legs to return to the starting position. Exhale at the end of the movement.

As with the barbell squat, this exercise works mainly the quadriceps and gluteus maximus. It is an excellent warm-up that can serve as training before passing onto a squat with weights. Series of 10 to 20 repetitions with a controlled movement provide good results.

Variation
To increase the intensity of the exercise it is possible to stop for two to five seconds at the horizontal thigh position.

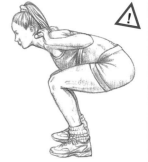

Whether the exercise be performed with a staff or a barbell, it is important to avoid any risk of injury at the lumbar level; never round the back.

SQUATS WITH LEGS APART

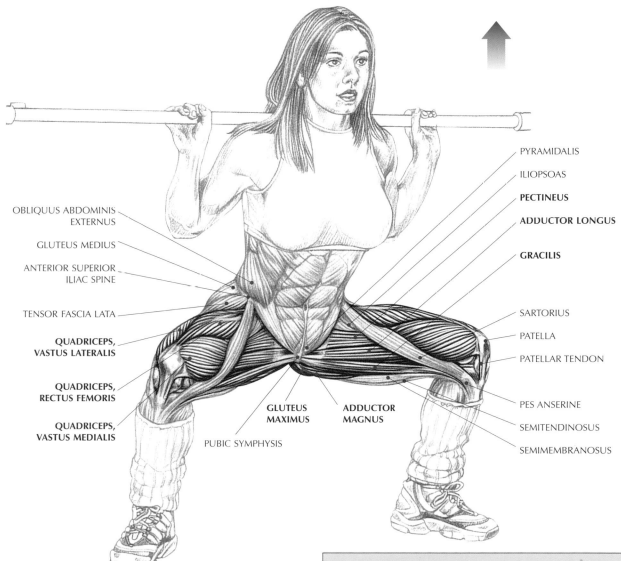

OBLIQUUS ABDOMINIS EXTERNUS

GLUTEUS MEDIUS

ANTERIOR SUPERIOR ILIAC SPINE

TENSOR FASCIA LATA

QUADRICEPS, VASTUS LATERALIS

QUADRICEPS, RECTUS FEMORIS

QUADRICEPS, VASTUS MEDIALIS

PUBIC SYMPHYSIS

GLUTEUS MAXIMUS

ADDUCTOR MAGNUS

PYRAMIDALIS

ILIOPSOAS

PECTINEUS

ADDUCTOR LONGUS

GRACILIS

SARTORIUS

PATELLA

PATELLAR TENDON

PES ANSERINE

SEMITENDINOSUS

SEMIMEMBRANOSUS

This movement is performed in the same way as the classic squat, but the legs are spread wide apart and the toes are pointed outward, which works the interior of the thighs intensely.

The muscle that are engaged are
* the quadriceps,
* the adductor group (the adductor magnus, adductor longus, adductor brevis, and adductor minimus), the pectineus and gracilis,
* the gluteal muscles,
* the hamstring muscles,
* the abdominals, and
* the lumbosacral group.

Note
The more the legs are bent, the less the back will be tilted forward.

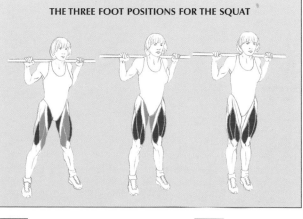

THE THREE FOOT POSITIONS FOR THE SQUAT

MUSCLES VERY ENGAGED

MUSCLES ENGAGED

4   SQUATS WITH A BAR IN FRONT

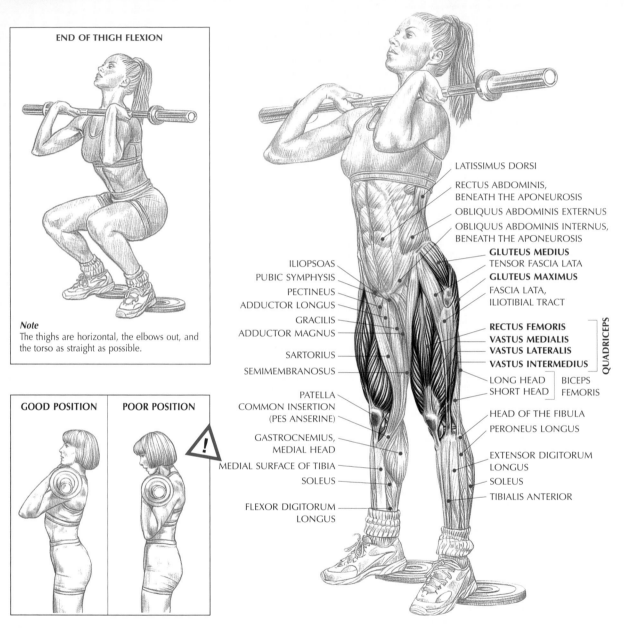

END OF THIGH FLEXION

Note
The thighs are horizontal, the elbows out, and the torso as straight as possible.

GOOD POSITION | **POOR POSITION**

LATISSIMUS DORSI

RECTUS ABDOMINIS, BENEATH THE APONEUROSIS

OBLIQUUS ABDOMINIS EXTERNUS

OBLIQUUS ABDOMINIS INTERNUS, BENEATH THE APONEUROSIS

GLUTEUS MEDIUS
TENSOR FASCIA LATA

GLUTEUS MAXIMUS

FASCIA LATA, ILIOTIBIAL TRACT

RECTUS FEMORIS
VASTUS MEDIALIS
VASTUS LATERALIS
VASTUS INTERMEDIUS

QUADRICEPS

LONG HEAD | BICEPS
SHORT HEAD | FEMORIS

HEAD OF THE FIBULA
PERONEUS LONGUS

EXTENSOR DIGITORUM LONGUS
SOLEUS
TIBIALIS ANTERIOR

ILIOPSOAS
PUBIC SYMPHYSIS
PECTINEUS
ADDUCTOR LONGUS
GRACILIS
ADDUCTOR MAGNUS

SARTORIUS
SEMIMEMBRANOSUS

PATELLA
COMMON INSERTION (PES ANSERINE)

GASTROCNEMIUS, MEDIAL HEAD
MEDIAL SURFACE OF TIBIA
SOLEUS

FLEXOR DIGITORUM LONGUS

Stand with the feet more or less shoulder width apart, grasp the bar in an overhand grip, and rest it on the upper pectoral muscles. So that the bar does not slide forward, it is important to push out the chest well and to raise the elbows as high as possible.

Take in a deep breath to maintain intrathoracic pressure, which prevents the torso from collapsing forward, arch the back slightly, contract the abdominal muscles, and flex the thighs until horizontal. Return to the initial position, breathing out at the end of the movement.

The bar placed anteriorly does not allow for any forward flexion of the torso, so the back will always be very straight. For easier execution a lift may be placed under the heels.

This type of squat puts a greater part of the effort onto the quadriceps; it is always worked with less weight than the classic squat. In the complete movement it engages the gluteal muscles, the hamstrings, the abdominal muscles, and the erector muscles of the spine.

Warning
To avoid nodding and falling forward it is essential when performing the bar squat to keep the elbows raised as high as possible, to push out the chest, and to curve the back slightly.

SQUATS WITH AN ELASTIC BAND

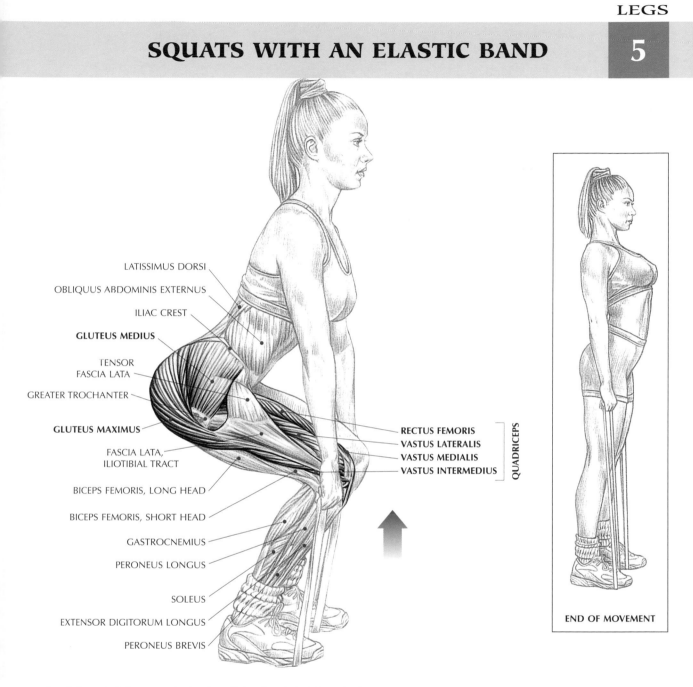

LATISSIMUS DORSI

OBLIQUUS ABDOMINIS EXTERNUS

ILIAC CREST

GLUTEUS MEDIUS

TENSOR
FASCIA LATA

GREATER TROCHANTER

GLUTEUS MAXIMUS

FASCIA LATA,
ILIOTIBIAL TRACT

BICEPS FEMORIS, LONG HEAD

BICEPS FEMORIS, SHORT HEAD

GASTROCNEMIUS

PERONEUS LONGUS

SOLEUS

EXTENSOR DIGITORUM LONGUS

PERONEUS BREVIS

RECTUS FEMORIS
VASTUS LATERALIS
VASTUS MEDIALIS
VASTUS INTERMEDIUS

QUADRICEPS

END OF MOVEMENT

Stand with legs slightly apart, the back well fixed and slightly arched. Bend the legs until the thighs are horizontal. Grab the elastic bands under each foot in an overhand grip with extended arms. Inhale and hold the breath; contract the stomach muscles and the lumbar area and extend the legs until standing. Exhale at the end of the movement. Return to the bent leg position without rounding the back and begin again.

This exercise mainly works the quadriceps and gluteal muscles, and to a lesser degree the erector muscles of the spine. Depending on the tension of the elastic bands, series of 10 to 20 repetitions provide good results.

Note
Unlike other thigh flexion movements, in which the hardest phase is at the beginning of leg extension, in the squat with elastic bands the hardest phase is at the extension of the legs, when the tension of the elastic bands is greatest.

Variation
It is possible to engage the superior part of the trapezius muscles by performing shoulder shrugs when the torso is vertical at the end of the movement.

6 ANTERIOR SQUATS WITH A STAFF

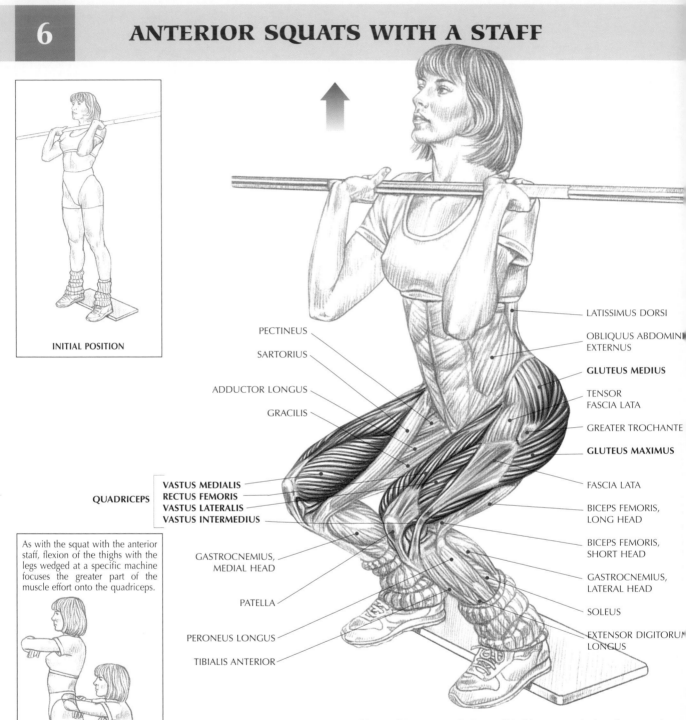

INITIAL POSITION

As with the squat with the anterior staff, flexion of the thighs with the legs wedged at a specific machine focuses the greater part of the muscle effort onto the quadriceps.

LATISSIMUS DORSI

OBLIQUUS ABDOMIN
EXTERNUS

GLUTEUS MEDIUS

TENSOR
FASCIA LATA

GREATER TROCHANTE

GLUTEUS MAXIMUS

FASCIA LATA

BICEPS FEMORIS,
LONG HEAD

BICEPS FEMORIS,
SHORT HEAD

GASTROCNEMIUS,
LATERAL HEAD

SOLEUS

EXTENSOR DIGITORUM
LONGUS

PECTINEUS

SARTORIUS

ADDUCTOR LONGUS

GRACILIS

QUADRICEPS
VASTUS MEDIALIS
RECTUS FEMORIS
VASTUS LATERALIS
VASTUS INTERMEDIUS

GASTROCNEMIUS,
MEDIAL HEAD

PATELLA

PERONEUS LONGUS

TIBIALIS ANTERIOR

Stand with the feet more or less shoulder width apart, with the staff held in an underhand grip and resting on the upper part of the pectoral and anterior deltoid muscles. Push out the chest and arch the back slightly. Inhale and flex the thighs. When they are horizontal, return to the initial position. Exhale at the end of the rise.

For perfect execution of the movement it is important to raise the elbows well. For better balance and to avoid lifting the heels off, it is possible to put a wedge under the heels. This exercise mainly works the quadriceps; it works the gluteus maximus a little less intensely.

Variation
The squat with a staff is an excellent movement for learning and becoming comfortable with performing thigh flexions before moving on to working with a barbell.

SQUATS AT A FRAME GUIDE

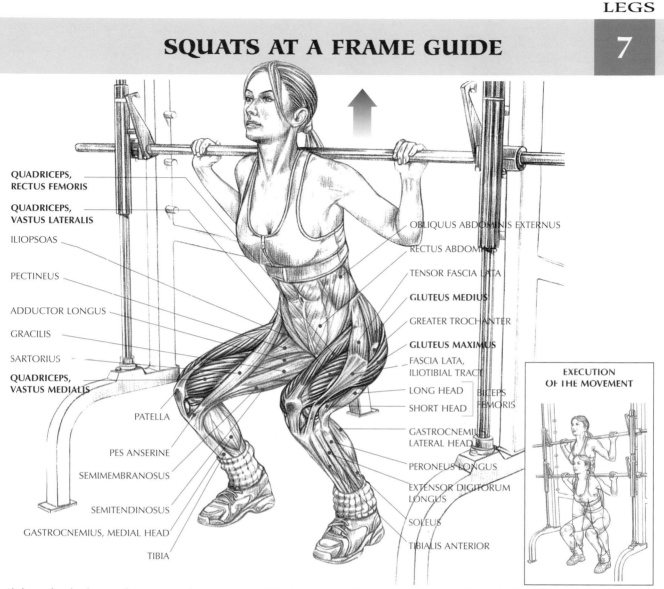

QUADRICEPS, RECTUS FEMORIS
QUADRICEPS, VASTUS LATERALIS
ILIOPSOAS
PECTINEUS
ADDUCTOR LONGUS
GRACILIS
SARTORIUS
QUADRICEPS, VASTUS MEDIALIS
PATELLA
PES ANSERINE
SEMIMEMBRANOSUS
SEMITENDINOSUS
GASTROCNEMIUS, MEDIAL HEAD
TIBIA

OBLIQUUS ABDOMINIS EXTERNUS
RECTUS ABDOMINIS
TENSOR FASCIA LATA
GLUTEUS MEDIUS
GREATER TROCHANTER
GLUTEUS MAXIMUS
FASCIA LATA, ILIOTIBIAL TRACT
LONG HEAD
SHORT HEAD
BICEPS FEMORIS
GASTROCNEMIUS LATERAL HEAD
PERONEUS LONGUS
EXTENSOR DIGITORUM LONGUS
SOLEUS
TIBIALIS ANTERIOR

EXECUTION OF THE MOVEMENT

Slide under the bar until it rests on the trapezius a little higher than the posterior deltoids. Grasp the bar firmly with both hands. Place the feet under the bar more or less greater than shoulder width apart. Pull the elbows backward; take a deep breath (to maintain an intrathoracic pressure, which will prevent the chest from collapsing forward); arch the back slightly by tilting the pelvis forward; contract the abdominal muscles; look straight ahead; lift the bar off the support stand, and don't forget to remove the lateral safety catches.

Crouch and control the descent without ever rounding the back to avoid all trauma. When the thighs are horizontal, extend the legs to end up in the initial position. Exhale at the end of the movement.

Variations
- When the feet are placed under the bar at the beginning, the muscles of the quadriceps and the gluteus maximus are mainly worked.
- Placing the feet in front of the bar limits flexion of the hip on lowering, and therefore the angle of the torso, which places part of the effort onto the quadriceps while limiting the work of the gluteus maximus. When the squat is performed with the feet spread apart, the adductor muscles of the thigh and the vastus lateralis of the quadriceps are engaged more intensely.

Note
No matter how the guided squat is performed it avoids excessive flexion of the torso, which limits the danger of injury in case of poor control of the movement.

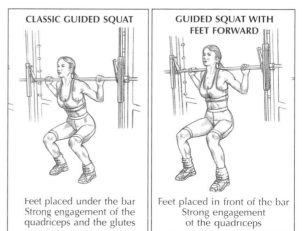

CLASSIC GUIDED SQUAT
Feet placed under the bar
Strong engagement of the quadriceps and the glutes

GUIDED SQUAT WITH FEET FORWARD
Feet placed in front of the bar
Strong engagement of the quadriceps

8 THIGH FLEXIONS IN A ROMAN CHAIR

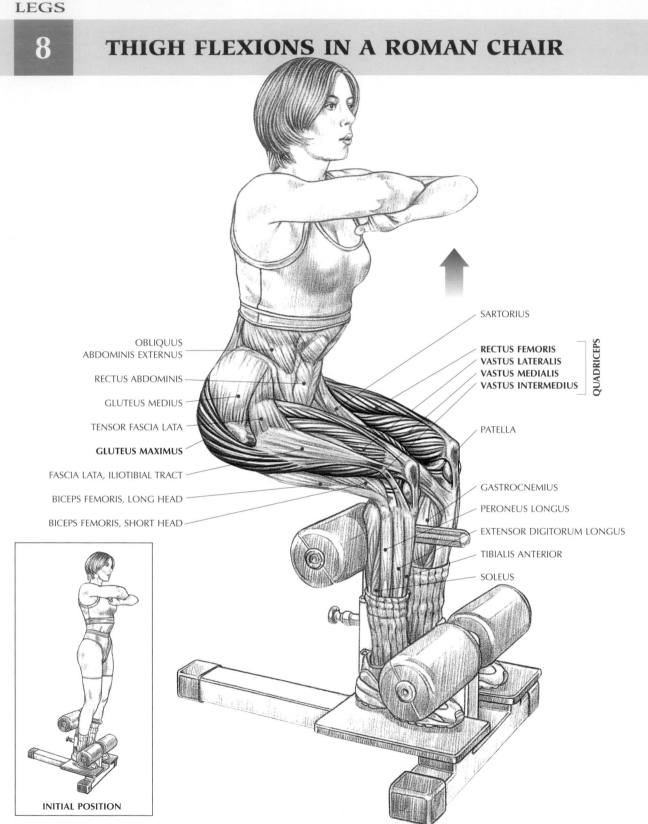

OBLIQUUS ABDOMINIS EXTERNUS

RECTUS ABDOMINIS

GLUTEUS MEDIUS

TENSOR FASCIA LATA

GLUTEUS MAXIMUS

FASCIA LATA, ILIOTIBIAL TRACT

BICEPS FEMORIS, LONG HEAD

BICEPS FEMORIS, SHORT HEAD

SARTORIUS

RECTUS FEMORIS
VASTUS LATERALIS
VASTUS MEDIALIS
VASTUS INTERMEDIUS

QUADRICEPS

PATELLA

GASTROCNEMIUS

PERONEUS LONGUS

EXTENSOR DIGITORUM LONGUS

TIBIALIS ANTERIOR

SOLEUS

INITIAL POSITION

Stand with the arms crossed in front, the feet wedged under the pads of the machine, and the back arched slightly. Inhale and slowly flex the thighs while thinking about keeping the torso vertical. When the femurs reach the horizontal position, extend the legs to return to the initial position. Exhale at the end of the effort.

Performing the squat at the roman chair eliminates bending of the torso, which reduces the work of gluteus maximus and focuses part of the effort onto the lower part of the quadriceps.

THIGH FLEXIONS WITH DUMBBELLS

INITIAL POSITION

LATISSIMUS DORSI

OBLIQUUS ABDOMINIS EXTERNUS

ILIAC CREST

TENSOR FASCIA LATA

GLUTEUS MEDIUS

GREATER TROCHANTER

GLUTEUS MAXIMUS

FASCIA LATA

BICEPS FEMORIS, LONG HEAD

BICEPS FEMORIS, SHORT HEAD

QUADRICEPS
RECTUS FEMORIS
VASTUS LATERALIS
VASTUS INTERMEDIUS
PATELLA
PERONEUS LONGUS
EXTENSOR DIGITORUM LONGUS

ADAPTATION OF THE BIPED

CHIMPANZEE

HUMAN

Stand, feet slightly apart, with a dumbbell in each hand, arms relaxed. Look straight ahead and inhale; arch the back slightly and flex the thighs. When the femurs reach horizontal, extend the legs to return to the initial position. Exhale at the end of the effort.

This exercise mainly works the quadriceps and the gluteal muscles.

Note
There is no point working with heavy weights; working with lighter weights and in series of 15 to 20 repetitions gives the best results.

In the chimpanzee, our closest relative, the big chest size associated with a not-well-developed gluteus maximus makes erecting the trunk difficult and makes for poor quality biped gait. The human is the only primate completely adapted to biped displacement.

Besides the significant development of the gluteus maximus, the whole human structure is adapted for bipedal existence. Thus, the size of the torso is decreased, which helps in straightening it, and unlike the gorilla or the chimpanzee, humans have the ability to keep the knee extended, which has made the standing position easy to maintain.

10 THIGH FLEXIONS

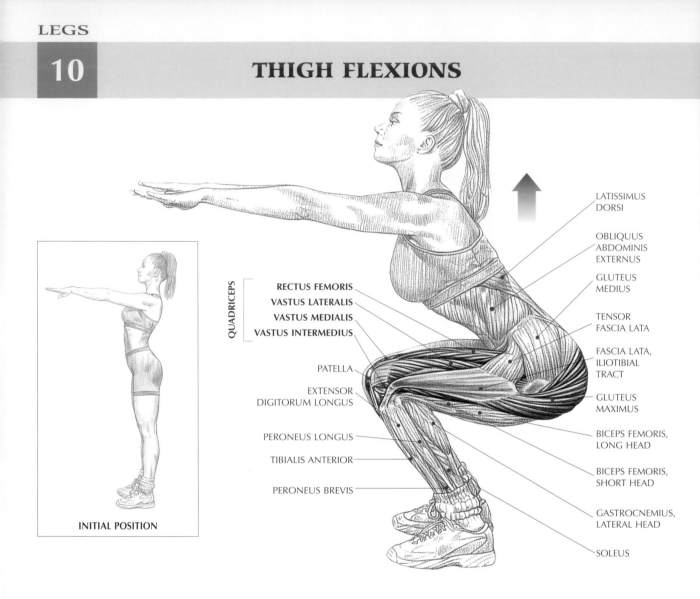

QUADRICEPS
- RECTUS FEMORIS
- VASTUS LATERALIS
- VASTUS MEDIALIS
- VASTUS INTERMEDIUS

PATELLA

EXTENSOR DIGITORUM LONGUS

PERONEUS LONGUS

TIBIALIS ANTERIOR

PERONEUS BREVIS

LATISSIMUS DORSI

OBLIQUUS ABDOMINIS EXTERNUS

GLUTEUS MEDIUS

TENSOR FASCIA LATA

FASCIA LATA, ILIOTIBIAL TRACT

GLUTEUS MAXIMUS

BICEPS FEMORIS, LONG HEAD

BICEPS FEMORIS, SHORT HEAD

GASTROCNEMIUS, LATERAL HEAD

SOLEUS

INITIAL POSITION

Stand with arms extended, feet slightly apart, head very straight, chest out, and back slightly arched. Inhale and crouch. When the thighs are horizontal, extend the legs by straightening the torso back to the initial position. Exhale at the end of the effort.

This exercise works mainly on the quadriceps and the gluteals. It is important to master the descending part and to perform the movement without jerking. The back must be very straight and the heels must not lift off the floor. As in all work without additional weights, long series of 15 to 20 repetitions provide the best results.

Variations

- The movement may be performed with the arms crossed or hanging at the sides of the body.
- Isometric contraction of the thighs may be maintained at the horizontal position for a few seconds. Stand with the feet slightly apart, arms horizontal and extended in front. Look straight ahead, chest out. Inhale, arch the back slightly, and flex the thighs. When the thighs reach horizontal, extend the legs to return to the initial position. Exhale at the end of the movement. This exercise works mainly the quadriceps and gluteal muscles.
- It is possible to perform the flexion by varying the arm positions, with either
  – the arms crossed in front or
  – the arms alongside the body.
- For people with stiff ankles or long femurs, a block placed underneath the heels can help to avoid too much tilt of the torso and anterior imbalance. This variation places part of the work onto the quadriceps. This is an excellent warm-up for the lower part of the body; it is also a very good beginner exercise to become familiar with flexion of the thighs before moving on to squat work.

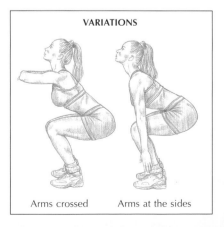

VARIATIONS

Arms crossed   Arms at the sides

THIGH FLEXIONS WITH LEGS APART

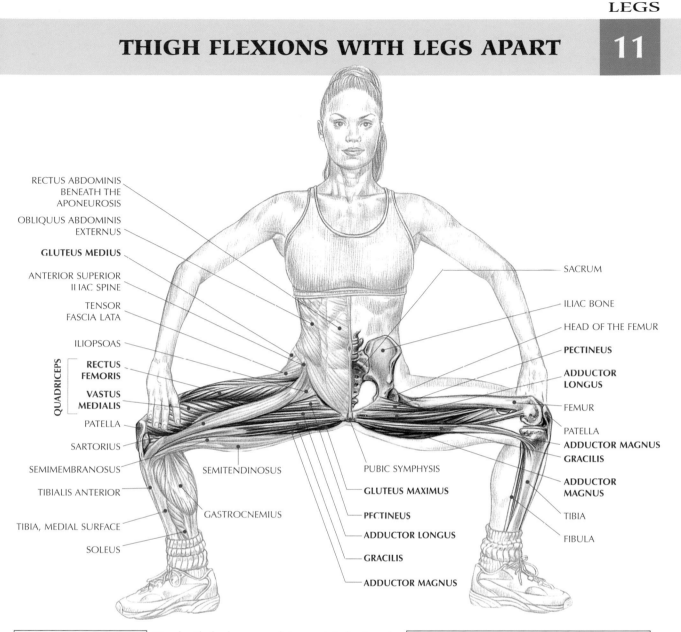

RECTUS ABDOMINIS BENEATH THE APONEUROSIS

OBLIQUUS ABDOMINIS EXTERNUS

GLUTEUS MEDIUS

ANTERIOR SUPERIOR ILIAC SPINE

TENSOR FASCIA LATA

ILIOPSOAS

QUADRICEPS
- **RECTUS FEMORIS**
- **VASTUS MEDIALIS**

PATELLA

SARTORIUS

SEMIMEMBRANOSUS

TIBIALIS ANTERIOR

TIBIA, MEDIAL SURFACE

SOLEUS

SEMITENDINOSUS

GASTROCNEMIUS

PUBIC SYMPHYSIS

GLUTEUS MAXIMUS

PECTINEUS

ADDUCTOR LONGUS

GRACILIS

ADDUCTOR MAGNUS

SACRUM

ILIAC BONE

HEAD OF THE FEMUR

PECTINEUS

ADDUCTOR LONGUS

FEMUR

PATELLA

ADDUCTOR MAGNUS
GRACILIS

ADDUCTOR MAGNUS

TIBIA

FIBULA

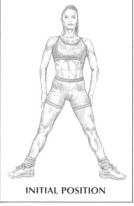

INITIAL POSITION

Stand with the legs spread, toes pointed outward, the back very straight, chest out. Inhale and flex the thighs until horizontal. Return to the initial position, exhaling at the end of the effort.

This exercise is performed slowly while trying to concentrate on feeling the muscle and contracting the buttocks muscles tightly at the end of straightening up. It is possible at the end of thigh flexion to maintain the horizontal position with an isometric contraction for a few seconds. As with all movements using the weight of the body, results are really only obtained in series. Thus it is recommended to effect several series of at least 20 repetitions until feeling a burn.

The solicited muscles are the quadriceps—predominantly the vastus lateralis and the adductor group (the adductor magnus, medius, and brevis; the pectineus; and the gracilis)—the gluteals (minimus, medius, and maximus), and the small external rotators of the thigh, located deep to the gluteals.

VARIATIONS

The movement can be performed with a staff on the shoulders, which has the effect of straightening the back, or with a staff held in front, sliding the staff along the tibias and thighs.

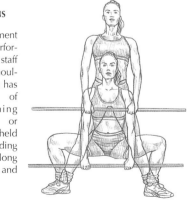

These two variations help limit torso movement and focus the effort on the lower extremity.

12 ALTERNATING LATERAL LUNGES

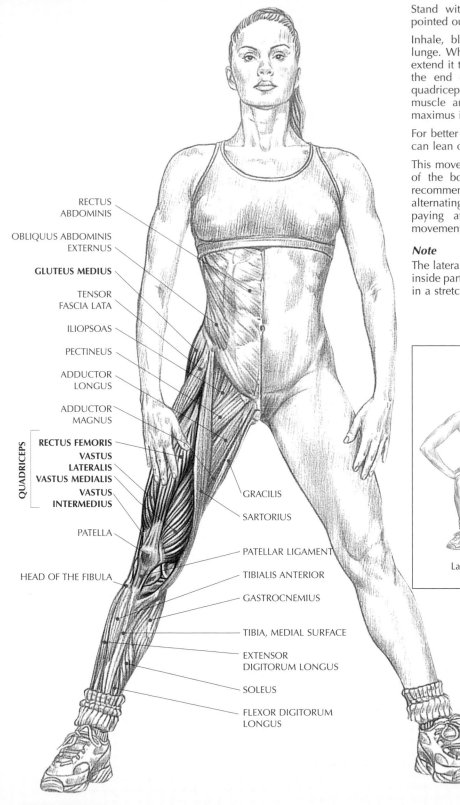

RECTUS
ABDOMINIS

OBLIQUUS ABDOMINIS
EXTERNUS

GLUTEUS MEDIUS

TENSOR
FASCIA LATA

ILIOPSOAS

PECTINEUS

ADDUCTOR
LONGUS

ADDUCTOR
MAGNUS

QUADRICEPS
RECTUS FEMORIS
VASTUS
LATERALIS
VASTUS MEDIALIS
VASTUS
INTERMEDIUS

PATELLA

HEAD OF THE FIBULA

GRACILIS

SARTORIUS

PATELLAR LIGAMENT

TIBIALIS ANTERIOR

GASTROCNEMIUS

TIBIA, MEDIAL SURFACE

EXTENSOR
DIGITORUM LONGUS

SOLEUS

FLEXOR DIGITORUM
LONGUS

Stand with the legs spread slightly apart, toes pointed outward.

Inhale, block the breath, and perform a lateral lunge. When the flexed thigh reaches horizontal, extend it to return to the initial position. Exhale at the end of extension. This exercise works the quadriceps, with preference on the lower part of the muscle and on the vastus lateralis; the gluteus maximus is also strongly solicited.

For better balance and to help the movement you can lean on the flexed leg.

This movement places a greater part of the weight of the body onto one leg, which is why it is recommended to work in series of 20 repetitions, alternating 10 on the right leg and 10 on the left, paying attention to perfect execution of the movement to protect the knee joints.

Note
The lateral lunge is also an excellent stretch for the inside part of the thigh. For this it could be included in a stretching program.

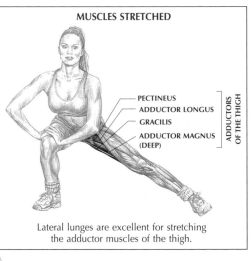

MUSCLES STRETCHED

PECTINEUS
ADDUCTOR LONGUS
GRACILIS
ADDUCTOR MAGNUS
(DEEP)

ADDUCTORS
OF THE THIGH

Lateral lunges are excellent for stretching
the adductor muscles of the thigh.

FLEXIONS ON ONE LEG

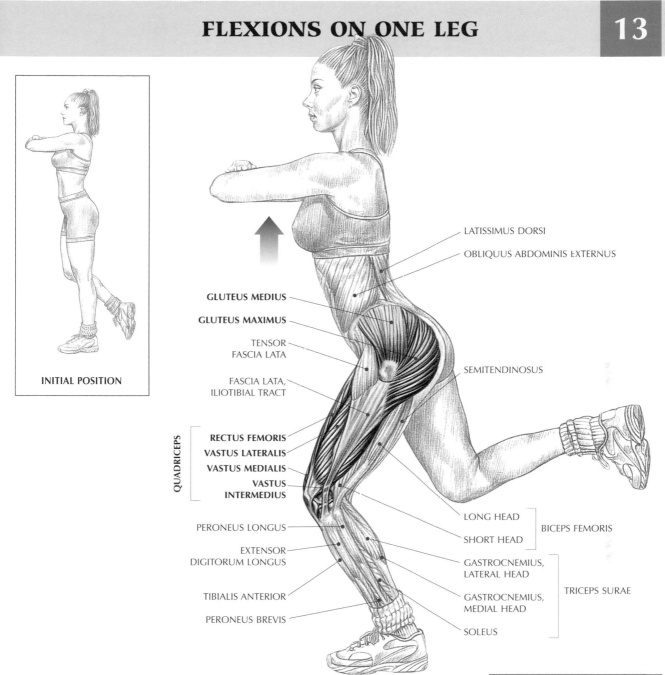

13

INITIAL POSITION

LATISSIMUS DORSI

OBLIQUUS ABDOMINIS EXTERNUS

GLUTEUS MEDIUS

GLUTEUS MAXIMUS

TENSOR FASCIA LATA

FASCIA LATA, ILIOTIBIAL TRACT

SEMITENDINOSUS

QUADRICEPS
RECTUS FEMORIS
VASTUS LATERALIS
VASTUS MEDIALIS
VASTUS INTERMEDIUS

PERONEUS LONGUS

EXTENSOR DIGITORUM LONGUS

TIBIALIS ANTERIOR

PERONEUS BREVIS

LONG HEAD

SHORT HEAD

BICEPS FEMORIS

GASTROCNEMIUS, LATERAL HEAD

GASTROCNEMIUS, MEDIAL HEAD

TRICEPS SURAE

SOLEUS

Stand on one leg with arms crossed in front, the other leg slightly bent behind. Inhale and perform a small flexion of the thigh; return to the initial position. Exhale at the end of the movement. This exercise is worked slowly, alternating long series on one side and then the other. The quadriceps and gluteus maximus are mainly solicited. This movement requires a sense of balance. As all the weight of the body is located on one leg and the articulation of the knee is relatively unstable in semiflexed position, do not overflex this articulation in order to maintain its integrity. Flexion on one leg is not for people with knee problems.

Variations

- To feel the work of the quadriceps, keep the knee slightly flexed without returning to the extended leg between each repetition.
- This movement can be performed bringing the nonstance leg forward.
- For more stability it is possible to work using a staff for support.

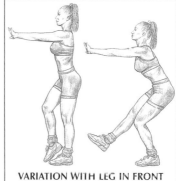

VARIATION WITH LEG IN FRONT

KNEE INSTABILITY

When the knee is in extension, the medial and lateral collateral ligaments stretch and prevent rotations of the articulation. Standing on one leg with the knee blocked in extension therefore does not require muscle activity to stabilize the articulation.

When the knee is flexed, the medial and lateral collateral ligaments are relaxed. In this position the articulation is only stabilized by the action of the muscles.

In flexion-rotation of the knee, the meniscus moves forward on the side of the rotation. If the extension of the articulation that follows is poorly controlled, the meniscus may not return to its place fast enough. It is then pinched between the condyles, which may lead to a relatively serious meniscus lesion. If, at the moment of being pinched, a small piece of the meniscus is cut off, a surgical operation may be necessary to remove it.

When performing asymmetrical exercises, such as flexions of the thigh on one leg or anterior lunges, it is important to preserve the knee articulation by controlling the speed and the integrity of the movement to avoid any injury.

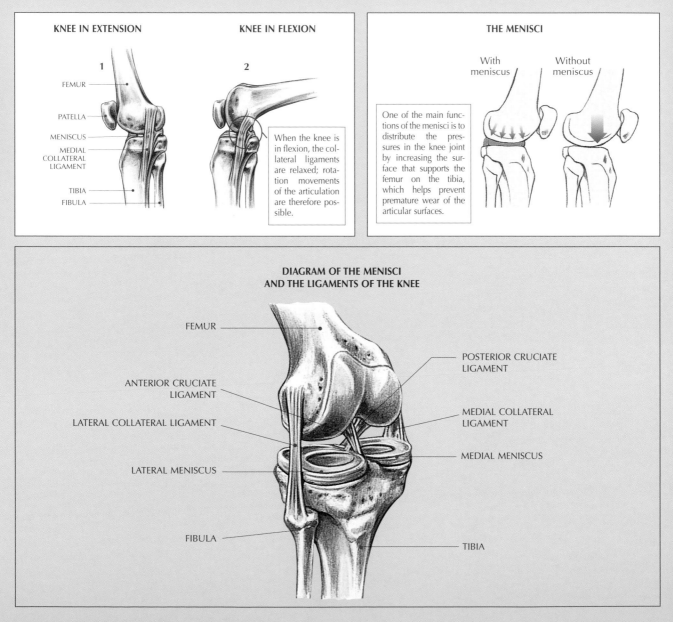

KNEE IN EXTENSION

KNEE IN FLEXION

1

2

FEMUR

PATELLA

MENISCUS

MEDIAL COLLATERAL LIGAMENT

TIBIA

FIBULA

When the knee is in flexion, the collateral ligaments are relaxed; rotation movements of the articulation are therefore possible.

THE MENISCI

With meniscus

Without meniscus

One of the main functions of the menisci is to distribute the pressures in the knee joint by increasing the surface that supports the femur on the tibia, which helps prevent premature wear of the articular surfaces.

DIAGRAM OF THE MENISCI AND THE LIGAMENTS OF THE KNEE

FEMUR

POSTERIOR CRUCIATE LIGAMENT

ANTERIOR CRUCIATE LIGAMENT

MEDIAL COLLATERAL LIGAMENT

LATERAL COLLATERAL LIGAMENT

MEDIAL MENISCUS

LATERAL MENISCUS

FIBULA

TIBIA

HACK SQUATS

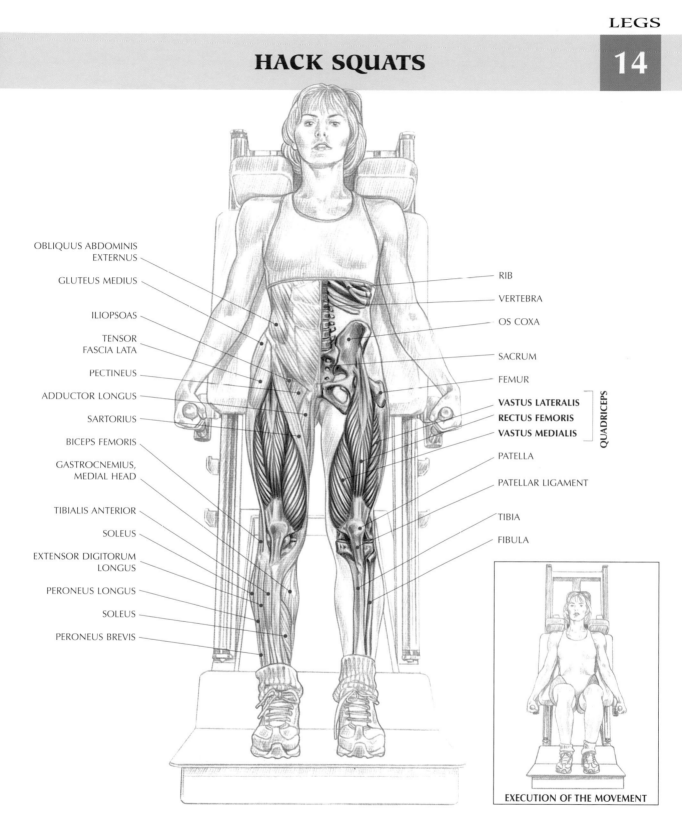

14

OBLIQUUS ABDOMINIS EXTERNUS

GLUTEUS MEDIUS

ILIOPSOAS

TENSOR FASCIA LATA

PECTINEUS

ADDUCTOR LONGUS

SARTORIUS

BICEPS FEMORIS

GASTROCNEMIUS, MEDIAL HEAD

TIBIALIS ANTERIOR

SOLEUS

EXTENSOR DIGITORUM LONGUS

PERONEUS LONGUS

SOLEUS

PERONEUS BREVIS

RIB

VERTEBRA

OS COXA

SACRUM

FEMUR

VASTUS LATERALIS
RECTUS FEMORIS
VASTUS MEDIALIS

QUADRICEPS

PATELLA

PATELLAR LIGAMENT

TIBIA

FIBULA

EXECUTION OF THE MOVEMENT

Position the body with knees bent, back against the backrest, shoulders wedged below the pads (*hack* means "yoke," the pads resembling the collar placed on draught animals), feet spread moderately apart. Inhale, release the catch, and flex the legs. Return to the initial position. Exhale at the end of the movement.

This movement places the effort onto the quadriceps. The more the legs are placed forward, the more the gluteals will be engaged, and the more the feet are spread apart, the more the adductors will be solicited. To protect the back, it is important to contract the abdominal muscles, which prevents lateral displacement of the pelvis and the spine.

15 THIGHS AT AN INCLINE PRESS

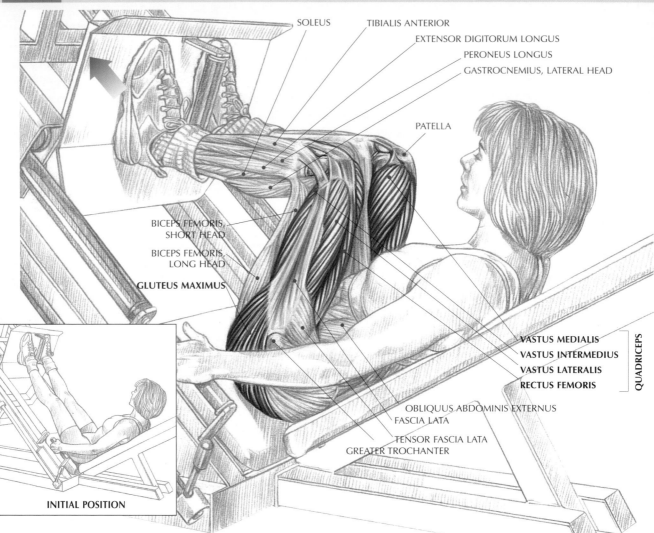

SOLEUS
TIBIALIS ANTERIOR
EXTENSOR DIGITORUM LONGUS
PERONEUS LONGUS
GASTROCNEMIUS, LATERAL HEAD

PATELLA

BICEPS FEMORIS, SHORT HEAD
BICEPS FEMORIS, LONG HEAD
GLUTEUS MAXIMUS

VASTUS MEDIALIS
VASTUS INTERMEDIUS
VASTUS LATERALIS
RECTUS FEMORIS

QUADRICEPS

OBLIQUUS ABDOMINIS EXTERNUS
FASCIA LATA
TENSOR FASCIA LATA
GREATER TROCHANTER

INITIAL POSITION

Position the body on the apparatus with the back wedged against the backrest, the feet moderately apart. Inhale, release the security catch, and flex the knees to the maximum so as to bring the thighs up against the rib cage. Return to the initial position, exhaling at the end of the movement.

If the feet are placed low on the platform, the quadriceps will be solicited in priority; if, however, the feet are raised toward the top of the platform, the effort will be more on the gluteals and the hamstrings. If the feet are spread apart, the effort will be directed more onto the adductors.

Note
This movement can be performed by people with back problems who cannot perform the squat; however, never remove the buttocks from the back support.

Warning
Using the press with heavy weights can cause displacement of the sacroiliac hinge in some people, which can lead to very painful muscle contractures.

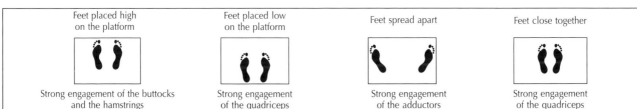

Feet placed high on the platform	Feet placed low on the platform	Feet spread apart	Feet close together
Strong engagement of the buttocks and the hamstrings	Strong engagement of the quadriceps	Strong engagement of the adductors	Strong engagement of the quadriceps

LIGAMENT HYPERLAXITY

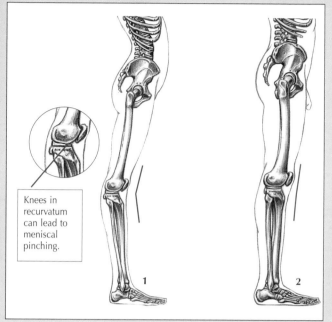

Warning

Reproduction in women often leads to hyperlax ligaments, a condition that allows for small displacements of the relatively immobile articulation of the pelvis (sacroiliac and pubic articulations) to facilitate the passage of the child during birthing.

This ligament hyperlaxity can lead to morphological details such as knees in recurvatum—that is to say, knees blocked in extension, which gives the impression that the leg is slightly flexed in the wrong direction.

Rarely pathological, knees in recurvatum can nevertheless lead to complications in some people, such as pinching of the menisci, which occurs when the knees move very quickly into extension and the menisci do not have time to slide, or during exercises for the thighs with heavy weights. For these reasons the instructor in group classes will recommend never completely extending the knees during exercises, and in exercises with additional weights, as in thigh presses or squats, will recommend never blocking the knee in extension.

It is good to remember that these caution recommendations only apply to people suffering from pathological recurvatum, most people can block the knees in extension without risk, the articulations stacking like the elements of the spinal column.

Knees in recurvatum can lead to meniscal pinching.

1. Typical female leg with recurvatum at the knee
2. Typical male leg with the articulations stacked like the elements of a column

LUXATION OF THE PATELLA

Quadriceps traction on the patella occurs in the axis of the body of the femur (that is to say, obliquely to the outside). The patella has a tendency to luxate laterally to the outside, but the lateral condyle of the femur is more prominent and prevents it from dislocating to the outside, and the traction of the inferior fibers of the vastus medialis of the quadriceps pull it back to medial.

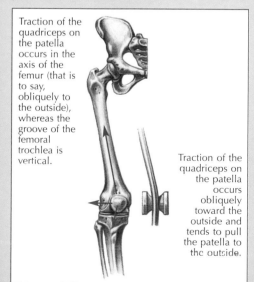

Traction of the quadriceps on the patella occurs in the axis of the femur (that is to say, obliquely to the outside), whereas the groove of the femoral trochlea is vertical.

Traction of the quadriceps on the patella occurs obliquely toward the outside and tends to pull the patella to the outside.

In women the greater obliquity of the femurs, a less prominent lateral condyle, and greater ligament laxity, along with a lack of tone in the inferior part of the medial and lateral vastae of the quadriceps, conspire for more frequent lateral luxation of the patella. Leg extension work is an excellent way to prevent this luxation as it reinforces the inferior part of the quadriceps, especially the medial vastae.

Note

Ligament laxity in women changes during the menstrual cycle and reaches its maximum during ovulation. It is thus during this period that the risk of injury at the level of the knee is greatest.

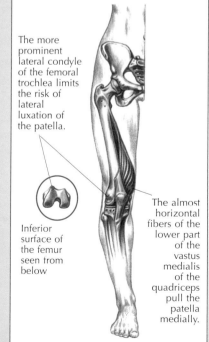

The more prominent lateral condyle of the femoral trochlea limits the risk of lateral luxation of the patella.

Inferior surface of the femur seen from below

The almost horizontal fibers of the lower part of the vastus medialis of the quadriceps pull the patella medially.

16

LEG EXTENSIONS
AT AN INCLINE MACHINE

INITIAL POSITION

OBLIQUUS ABDOMINIS EXTERNUS

RECTUS ABDOMINIS

ILIOPSOAS

PECTINEUS

ADDUCTOR LONGUS

SARTORIUS

QUADRICEPS, RECTUS FEMORIS

QUADRICEPS, VASTUS MEDIALIS

PATELLA

PATELLAR LIGAMENT

ANTERIOR SUPERIOR ILIAC SPINE

GLUTEUS MEDIUS

QUADRICEPS, VASTUS LATERALIS

TENSOR FASCIA LATA

FASCIA LATA

QUADRICEPS, VASTUS INTERMEDIUS

GLUTEUS MAXIMUS

TIBIALIS ANTERIOR

EXTENSOR DIGITORUM LONGUS

PERONEUS LONGUS

SOLEUS

If equipment is unavailable, it is possible to perform the extensions sitting in a chair. In this case the movement needs to be performed slowly, one leg after the other, concentrating on the muscle contraction at the end of extension.

Note

As with extensions at a machine, the more the torso is inclined posteriorly, the more the rectus femoris will be solicited.

Sit at the machine with the hands gripping the handles or the seat to immobilize the torso, knees flexed, ankles placed under the pads. Inhale and extend the legs to horizontal. Exhale at the end of the movement.

This is the best exercise to isolate the quadriceps. Note that the more the back is tilted, the more the pelvis will be in a posterior tilt. The rectus femoris, which is the midline biarticular portion of the quadriceps, will thus be stretched, intensifying its work in extension of the legs.

This exercise is recommended for beginners to develop enough strength before moving on to more advanced techniques.

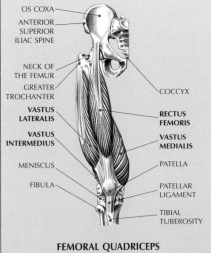

OS COXA

ANTERIOR SUPERIOR ILIAC SPINE

NECK OF THE FEMUR

GREATER TROCHANTER

VASTUS LATERALIS

VASTUS INTERMEDIUS

MENISCUS

FIBULA

COCCYX

RECTUS FEMORIS

VASTUS MEDIALIS

PATELLA

PATELLAR LIGAMENT

TIBIAL TUBEROSITY

FEMORAL QUADRICEPS

THIGH RAISES

LATISSIMUS DORSI

OBLIQUUS
ABDOMINIS EXTERNUS

GLUTEUS MEDIUS

TENSOR FASCIA LATA

FASCIA LATA,
ILIOTIBIAL TRACT

RECTUS FEMORIS

VASTUS LATERALIS

VASTUS MEDIALIS

VASTUS INTERMEDIUS

QUADRICEPS

PATELLA

BICEPS FEMORIS,
SHORT HEAD

SEMITENDINOSUS

GASTROCNEMIUS,
LATERAL HEAD

PERONEUS LONGUS

EXTENSOR
DIGITORUM LONGUS

TIBIALIS ANTERIOR

SOLEUS

PERONEUS BREVIS

GREATER TROCHANTER

BICEPS FEMORIS,
LONG HEAD

GLUTEUS MAXIMUS

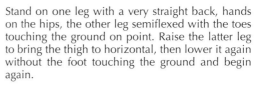

INITIAL POSITION

Stand on one leg with a very straight back, hands on the hips, the other leg semiflexed with the toes touching the ground on point. Raise the latter leg to bring the thigh to horizontal, then lower it again without the foot touching the ground and begin again.

This exercise works mainly the rectus femoris and the tensor fascia lata. All the other flexors of the hip (the iliopsoas, the sartorius, and the pectineus) are also solicited but less intensely.

For more effectiveness, it is recommended to raise the thigh tonically (that is, as quickly as possible) but to lower it back down slowly.

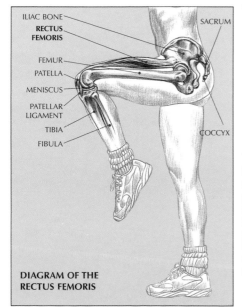

ILIAC BONE

**RECTUS
FEMORIS**

FEMUR

PATELLA

MENISCUS

PATELLAR
LIGAMENT

TIBIA

FIBULA

SACRUM

COCCYX

**DIAGRAM OF THE
RECTUS FEMORIS**

The rectus muscle of the thigh is the only portion of the quadriceps that is biarticular (that spans two joints); it spans the knee joint and the hip joint. The rectus muscle is therefore a powerful extensor of the lower leg, but it is also a powerful flexor of the hip, the action that this exercise addresses.

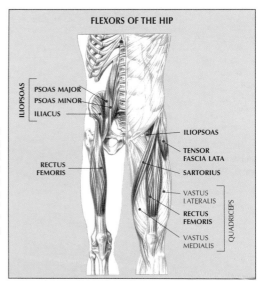

FLEXORS OF THE HIP

ILIOPSOAS

PSOAS MAJOR
PSOAS MINOR
ILIACUS

ILIOPSOAS

TENSOR
FASCIA LATA

SARTORIUS

RECTUS
FEMORIS

VASTUS
LATERALIS

**RECTUS
FEMORIS**

VASTUS
MEDIALIS

QUADRICEPS

18 THIGH RAISES WITH WEIGHTS

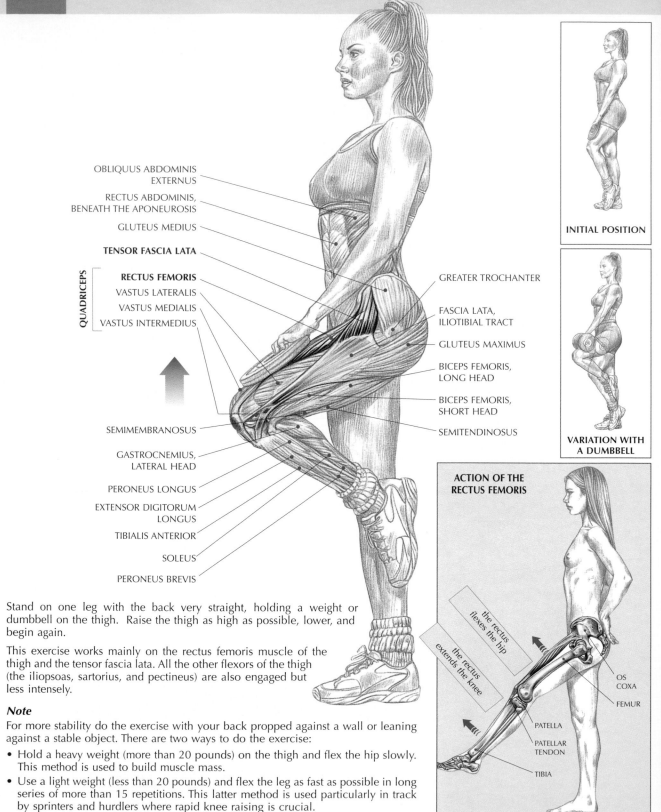

OBLIQUUS ABDOMINIS EXTERNUS

RECTUS ABDOMINIS, BENEATH THE APONEUROSIS

GLUTEUS MEDIUS

TENSOR FASCIA LATA

QUADRICEPS

RECTUS FEMORIS
VASTUS LATERALIS
VASTUS MEDIALIS
VASTUS INTERMEDIUS

SEMIMEMBRANOSUS

GASTROCNEMIUS, LATERAL HEAD

PERONEUS LONGUS

EXTENSOR DIGITORUM LONGUS

TIBIALIS ANTERIOR

SOLEUS

PERONEUS BREVIS

GREATER TROCHANTER

FASCIA LATA, ILIOTIBIAL TRACT

GLUTEUS MAXIMUS

BICEPS FEMORIS, LONG HEAD

BICEPS FEMORIS, SHORT HEAD

SEMITENDINOSUS

INITIAL POSITION

VARIATION WITH A DUMBBELL

ACTION OF THE RECTUS FEMORIS

the rectus flexes the hip

the rectus extends the knee

OS COXA

FEMUR

PATELLA

PATELLAR TENDON

TIBIA

Stand on one leg with the back very straight, holding a weight or dumbbell on the thigh. Raise the thigh as high as possible, lower, and begin again.

This exercise works mainly on the rectus femoris muscle of the thigh and the tensor fascia lata. All the other flexors of the thigh (the iliopsoas, sartorius, and pectineus) are also engaged but less intensely.

Note

For more stability do the exercise with your back propped against a wall or leaning against a stable object. There are two ways to do the exercise:

• Hold a heavy weight (more than 20 pounds) on the thigh and flex the hip slowly. This method is used to build muscle mass.
• Use a light weight (less than 20 pounds) and flex the leg as fast as possible in long series of more than 15 repetitions. This latter method is used particularly in track by sprinters and hurdlers where rapid knee raising is crucial.

ADDUCTORS ON THE FLOOR

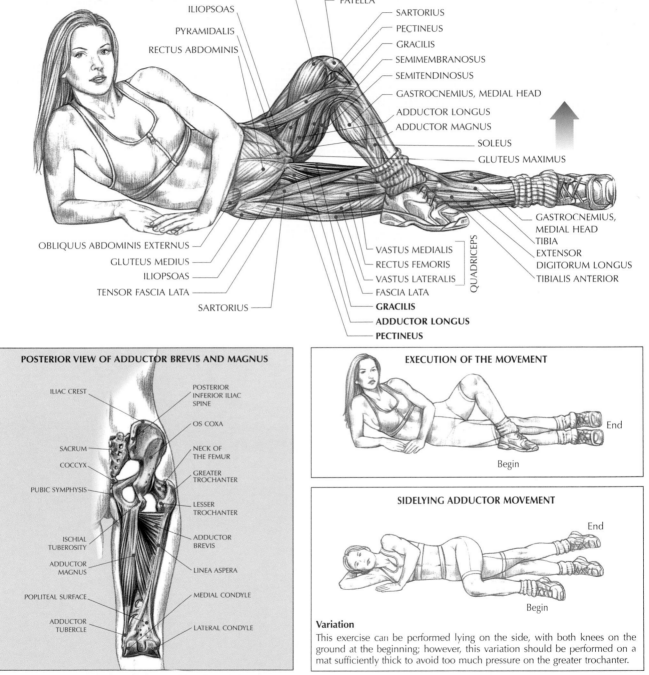

QUADRICEPS, VASTUS MEDIALIS
ILIOPSOAS
PYRAMIDALIS
RECTUS ABDOMINIS

PATELLA
SARTORIUS
PECTINEUS
GRACILIS
SEMIMEMBRANOSUS
SEMITENDINOSUS
GASTROCNEMIUS, MEDIAL HEAD
ADDUCTOR LONGUS
ADDUCTOR MAGNUS
SOLEUS
GLUTEUS MAXIMUS

GASTROCNEMIUS, MEDIAL HEAD
TIBIA
EXTENSOR DIGITORUM LONGUS
TIBIALIS ANTERIOR

OBLIQUUS ABDOMINIS EXTERNUS
GLUTEUS MEDIUS
ILIOPSOAS
TENSOR FASCIA LATA
SARTORIUS

VASTUS MEDIALIS
RECTUS FEMORIS
VASTUS LATERALIS
FASCIA LATA
GRACILIS
ADDUCTOR LONGUS
PECTINEUS

QUADRICEPS

POSTERIOR VIEW OF ADDUCTOR BREVIS AND MAGNUS

ILIAC CREST
SACRUM
COCCYX
PUBIC SYMPHYSIS
ISCHIAL TUBEROSITY
ADDUCTOR MAGNUS
POPLITEAL SURFACE
ADDUCTOR TUBERCLE

POSTERIOR INFERIOR ILIAC SPINE
OS COXA
NECK OF THE FEMUR
GREATER TROCHANTER
LESSER TROCHANTER
ADDUCTOR BREVIS
LINEA ASPERA
MEDIAL CONDYLE
LATERAL CONDYLE

EXECUTION OF THE MOVEMENT

End
Begin

SIDELYING ADDUCTOR MOVEMENT

End
Begin

Variation
This exercise can be performed lying on the side, with both knees on the ground at the beginning; however, this variation should be performed on a mat sufficiently thick to avoid too much pressure on the greater trochanter.

Lie on the side, leaning on the forearm with the leg on the floor extended, the other leg bent with the foot flat in front of the opposite knee. Raise the leg off the ground as high as possible. Maintain the contraction for two or three seconds and begin again.

Although the amplitude is greatly diminished, this movement nevertheless allows you to feel the working of the pectineus, adductor brevis, adductor minimus, and adductor longus muscles, with most of the effort on the adductor magnus and gracilis. Series of 10 to 20 repetitions executed slowly bring the best results. For variation, it's possible to sustain an isometric contraction of the raised leg for 10 seconds between each repetition.

20 ADDUCTORS AT A LOW PULLEY

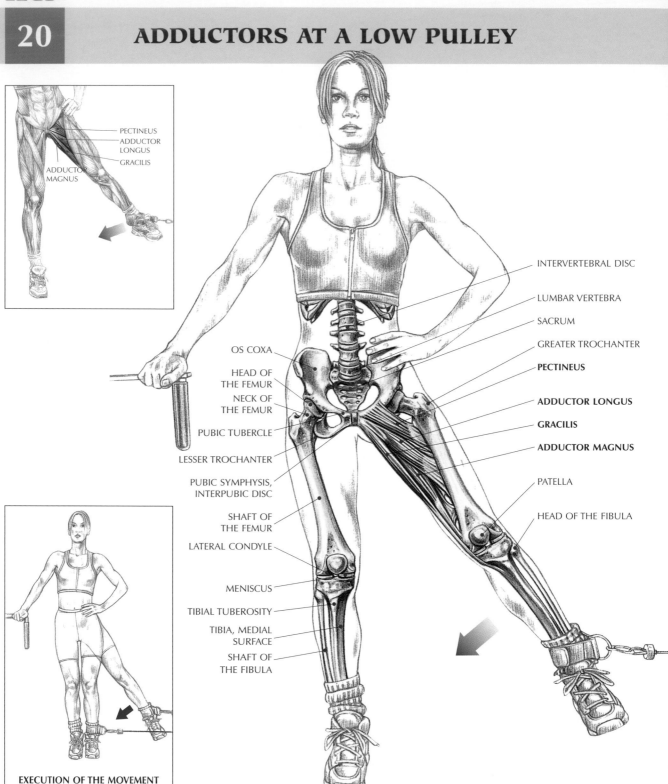

PECTINEUS
ADDUCTOR LONGUS
GRACILIS
ADDUCTOR MAGNUS

INTERVERTEBRAL DISC

LUMBAR VERTEBRA

SACRUM

GREATER TROCHANTER

PECTINEUS

ADDUCTOR LONGUS

GRACILIS

ADDUCTOR MAGNUS

PATELLA

HEAD OF THE FIBULA

OS COXA

HEAD OF THE FEMUR

NECK OF THE FEMUR

PUBIC TUBERCLE

LESSER TROCHANTER

PUBIC SYMPHYSIS, INTERPUBIC DISC

SHAFT OF THE FEMUR

LATERAL CONDYLE

MENISCUS

TIBIAL TUBEROSITY

TIBIA, MEDIAL SURFACE

SHAFT OF THE FIBULA

EXECUTION OF THE MOVEMENT

Stand on one leg with the cuff around the other ankle. The opposite hand is used for support on the frame of the machine or any other support. Bring the cuffed leg across in front of the support leg.

This exercise works the adductor group (pectineus; adductors brevis, minimus, longus, and magnus; and gracilis). It is excellent for definition on the inside of the thighs and is performed toward this end with long repetitions.

ADDUCTORS AT A MACHINE

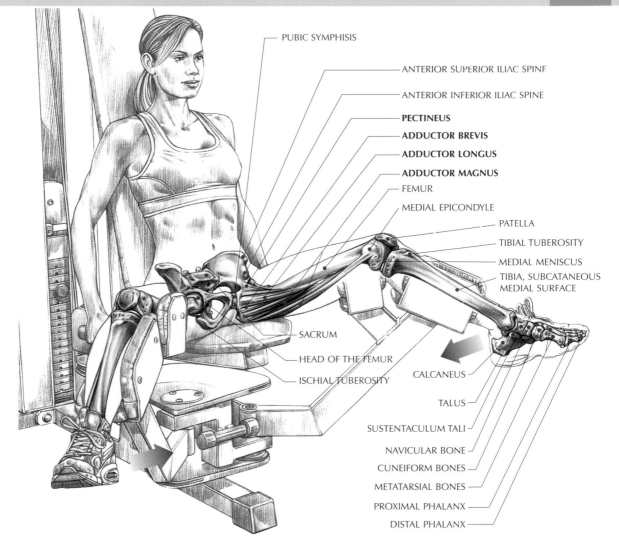

- PUBIC SYMPHISIS
- ANTERIOR SUPERIOR ILIAC SPINE
- ANTERIOR INFERIOR ILIAC SPINE
- **PECTINEUS**
- **ADDUCTOR BREVIS**
- **ADDUCTOR LONGUS**
- **ADDUCTOR MAGNUS**
- FEMUR
- MEDIAL EPICONDYLE
- PATELLA
- TIBIAL TUBEROSITY
- MEDIAL MENISCUS
- TIBIA, SUBCATANEOUS MEDIAL SURFACE
- SACRUM
- HEAD OF THE FEMUR
- ISCHIAL TUBEROSITY
- CALCANEUS
- TALUS
- SUSTENTACULUM TALI
- NAVICULAR BONE
- CUNEIFORM BONES
- METATARSIAL BONES
- PROXIMAL PHALANX
- DISTAL PHALANX

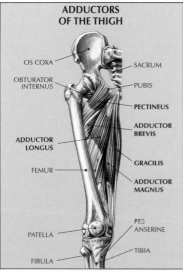

ADDUCTORS OF THE THIGH

- OS COXA
- OBTURATOR INTERNUS
- SACRUM
- PUBIS
- **PECTINEUS**
- **ADDUCTOR BREVIS**
- **ADDUCTOR LONGUS**
- **GRACILIS**
- FEMUR
- **ADDUCTOR MAGNUS**
- PATELLA
- PES ANSERINE
- TIBIA
- FIBULA

Sit at the machine with legs spread apart. Squeeze the thighs and return to the initial position with a controlled movement.

This exercise works the adductor muscle group of the thigh (pectineus; adductors brevis, magnus, and longus; and gracilis). It allows you to use heavier weights then adduction with a low cable, but its amplitude isn't as great. Long series performed until you feel a burn produce the best results.

Note

This movement can be performed to strengthen the adductors. This group of muscles is often the location for injuries of shortened muscles that are subjected to sudden effort. For this reason it is recommended to increase the resistance progressively and work in conjunction with a specific stretching program at the end of the session.

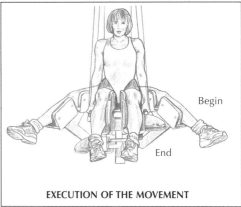

Begin

End

EXECUTION OF THE MOVEMENT

22 ADDUCTORS WITH A BALL

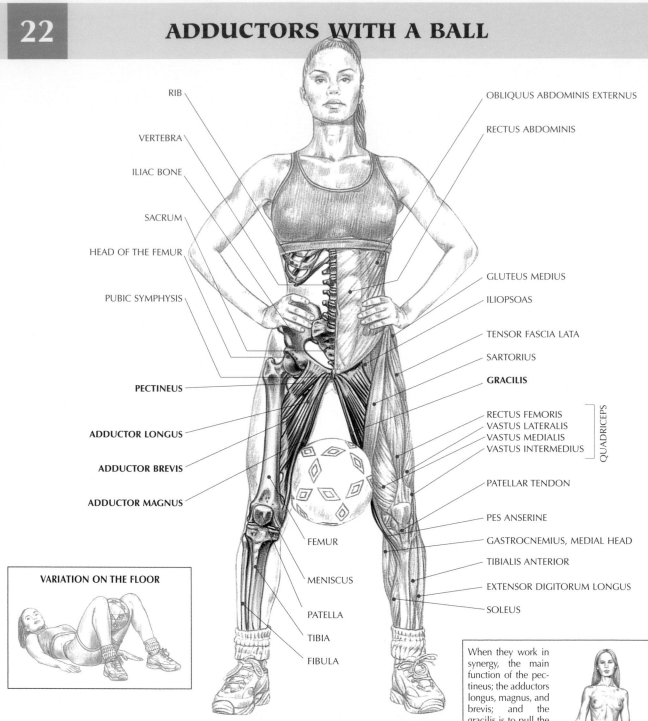

RIB

VERTEBRA

ILIAC BONE

SACRUM

HEAD OF THE FEMUR

PUBIC SYMPHYSIS

PECTINEUS

ADDUCTOR LONGUS

ADDUCTOR BREVIS

ADDUCTOR MAGNUS

FEMUR

MENISCUS

PATELLA

TIBIA

FIBULA

OBLIQUUS ABDOMINIS EXTERNUS

RECTUS ABDOMINIS

GLUTEUS MEDIUS

ILIOPSOAS

TENSOR FASCIA LATA

SARTORIUS

GRACILIS

RECTUS FEMORIS
VASTUS LATERALIS
VASTUS MEDIALIS
VASTUS INTERMEDIUS

QUADRICEPS

PATELLAR TENDON

PES ANSERINE

GASTROCNEMIUS, MEDIAL HEAD

TIBIALIS ANTERIOR

EXTENSOR DIGITORUM LONGUS

SOLEUS

VARIATION ON THE FLOOR

Stand with knees slightly bent with a ball placed between the legs. Squeeze the thighs as hard as possible, as if trying to pop the ball. Maintain the contraction a few seconds and begin again. Long series obtain the best results. You can also maintain a single contraction as long as possible. As in all movements without additional weights, to be really effective, this needs to be performed until you feel a burn.

This exercise works the adductor group, mainly the adductors brevis, longus, and magnus and the gracilis and to a lesser extent the pectineus.

Note
As there is little or no articular displacement during the muscle contraction (isometric work), this movement can be performed by people who suffer at the hips (coxofemoral joints).

When they work in synergy, the main function of the pectineus; the adductors longus, magnus, and brevis; and the gracilis is to pull the femur into adduction, flexion, and external rotation. For their powerful action of bringing the thighs together, the Romans called them the custodes virginitatis, the "protectors of virtue."

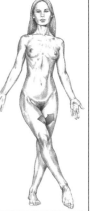

STIFF-LEGGED DEAD LIFTS

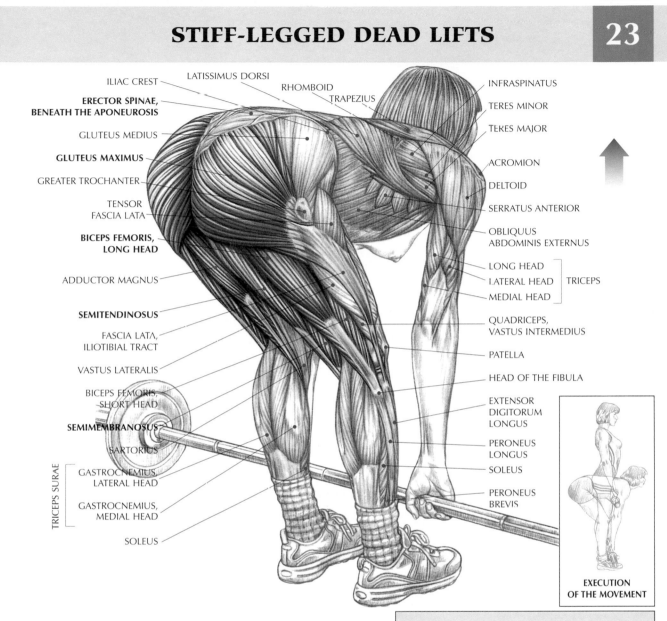

LATISSIMUS DORSI

ILIAC CREST

RHOMBOID

TRAPEZIUS

ERECTOR SPINAE, BENEATH THE APONEUROSIS

GLUTEUS MEDIUS

GLUTEUS MAXIMUS

GREATER TROCHANTER

TENSOR FASCIA LATA

BICEPS FEMORIS, LONG HEAD

ADDUCTOR MAGNUS

SEMITENDINOSUS

FASCIA LATA, ILIOTIBIAL TRACT

VASTUS LATERALIS

BICEPS FEMORIS, SHORT HEAD

SEMIMEMBRANOSUS

SARTORIUS

TRICEPS SURAE

GASTROCNEMIUS, LATERAL HEAD

GASTROCNEMIUS, MEDIAL HEAD

SOLEUS

INFRASPINATUS

TERES MINOR

TERES MAJOR

ACROMION

DELTOID

SERRATUS ANTERIOR

OBLIQUUS ABDOMINIS EXTERNUS

LONG HEAD

LATERAL HEAD

MEDIAL HEAD

TRICEPS

QUADRICEPS, VASTUS INTERMEDIUS

PATELLA

HEAD OF THE FIBULA

EXTENSOR DIGITORUM LONGUS

PERONEUS LONGUS

SOLEUS

PERONEUS BREVIS

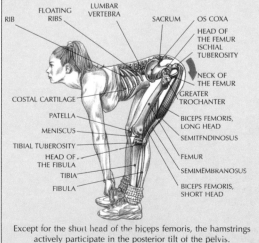

EXECUTION OF THE MOVEMENT

Stand with the feet slightly apart, facing the bar placed on the ground. Inhale, bending forward and keeping the back arched and, if possible, maintaining the legs in extension. Grasp the bar in an overhand grip, arms relaxed, and straighten the torso to vertical, with the back still fixed; the tilting occurs at the level of the hips. Exhale at the end of the movement. Return to the initial position, without replacing the bar, and begin again. It is important when executing the movement never to round the back to avoid all risk of injury.

This exercise solicits the spinal muscle group, the muscles located deep on each side of the vertebral column (or spine), whose main function is to straighten it up. In the straightening of the torso, during the antero-posterior tilt of the pelvis, the gluteus maximus and the hamstrings (with the exception of the short head of the biceps femoris) contribute strongly. The stiff-legged dead lift stretches the backs of the thighs during flexion. For a more effective stretch you may place the feet higher than the bar.

Note

When performed with very light weight, the stiff-legged dead lift can be considered as a stretch for the hamstrings. The greater the weight, the more the gluteals will take over from the hamstrings to right or straighten the pelvis.

RIB

FLOATING RIBS

LUMBAR VERTEBRA

SACRUM

OS COXA

HEAD OF THE FEMUR ISCHIAL TUBEROSITY

NECK OF THE FEMUR

GREATER TROCHANTER

BICEPS FEMORIS, LONG HEAD

SEMITENDINOSUS

FEMUR

SEMIMEMBRANOSUS

BICEPS FEMORIS, SHORT HEAD

COSTAL CARTILAGE

PATELLA

MENISCUS

TIBIAL TUBEROSITY

HEAD OF THE FIBULA

TIBIA

FIBULA

Except for the short head of the biceps femoris, the hamstrings actively participate in the posterior tilt of the pelvis.

GOOD MORNINGS

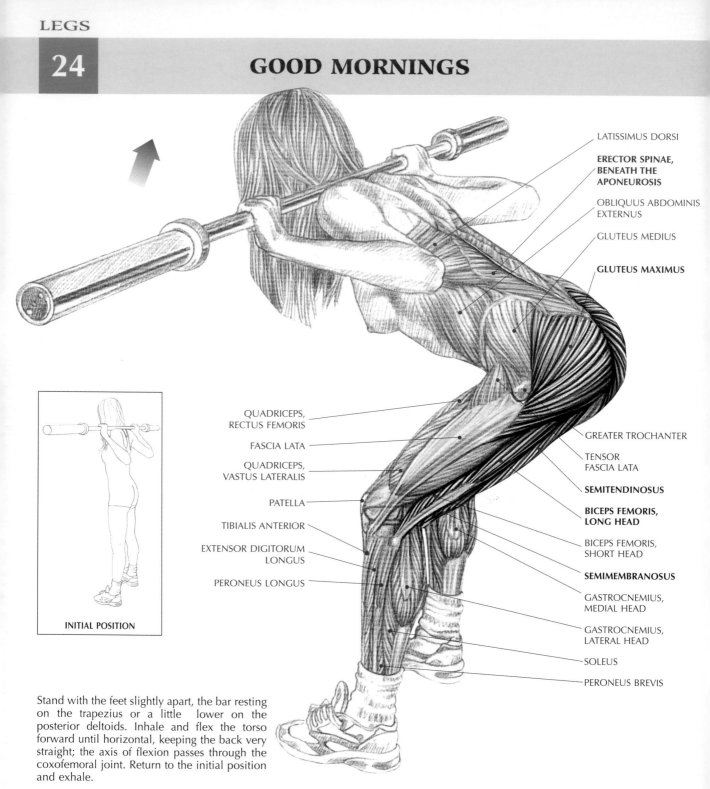

LATISSIMUS DORSI

**ERECTOR SPINAE,
BENEATH THE
APONEUROSIS**

OBLIQUUS ABDOMINIS
EXTERNUS

GLUTEUS MEDIUS

GLUTEUS MAXIMUS

GREATER TROCHANTER

TENSOR
FASCIA LATA

SEMITENDINOSUS

**BICEPS FEMORIS,
LONG HEAD**

BICEPS FEMORIS,
SHORT HEAD

SEMIMEMBRANOSUS

GASTROCNEMIUS,
MEDIAL HEAD

GASTROCNEMIUS,
LATERAL HEAD

SOLEUS

PERONEUS BREVIS

QUADRICEPS,
RECTUS FEMORIS

FASCIA LATA

QUADRICEPS,
VASTUS LATERALIS

PATELLA

TIBIALIS ANTERIOR

EXTENSOR DIGITORUM
LONGUS

PERONEUS LONGUS

INITIAL POSITION

Stand with the feet slightly apart, the bar resting on the trapezius or a little lower on the posterior deltoids. Inhale and flex the torso forward until horizontal, keeping the back very straight; the axis of flexion passes through the coxofemoral joint. Return to the initial position and exhale.

For easier execution you may flex the knees slightly.

This movement works gluteus maximus and the spinal group and is especially remarkable for its action on the hamstrings (with the exception of the short head of the biceps, which is only a leg flexor). Other than flexion at the knee, the hamstrings' main function is posterior tilting of the pelvis, straightening the torso if it is locked together by isometric contraction with the abdominal muscles and the lumbosacral muscles.

To feel the hamstrings better, never work with heavy weights. In the negative phase the good morning is excellent for stretching behind the thighs. When worked regularly it helps avoid injuries that may occur during the heavy squat.

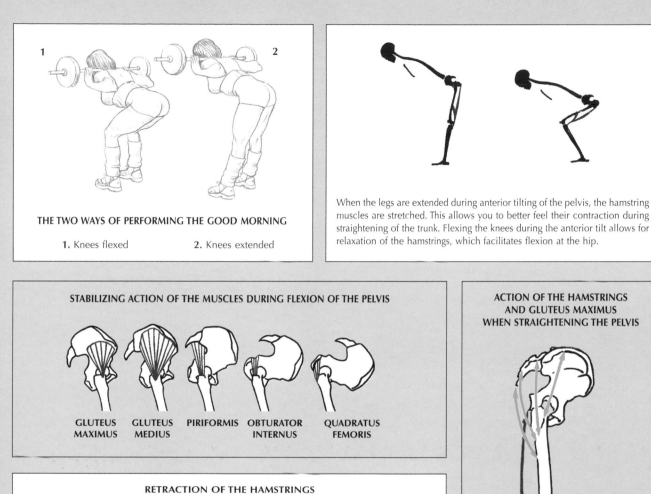

THE TWO WAYS OF PERFORMING THE GOOD MORNING

1. Knees flexed   **2.** Knees extended

When the legs are extended during anterior tilting of the pelvis, the hamstring muscles are stretched. This allows you to better feel their contraction during straightening of the trunk. Flexing the knees during the anterior tilt allows for relaxation of the hamstrings, which facilitates flexion at the hip.

STABILIZING ACTION OF THE MUSCLES DURING FLEXION OF THE PELVIS

| GLUTEUS MAXIMUS | GLUTEUS MEDIUS | PIRIFORMIS | OBTURATOR INTERNUS | QUADRATUS FEMORIS |

RETRACTION OF THE HAMSTRINGS

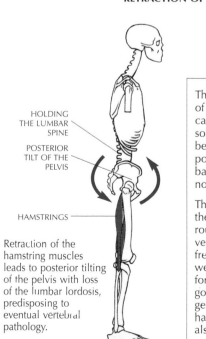

HOLDING THE LUMBAR SPINE

POSTERIOR TILT OF THE PELVIS

HAMSTRINGS

Retraction of the hamstring muscles leads to posterior tilting of the pelvis with loss of the lumbar lordosis, predisposing to eventual vertebral pathology.

The sitting posture we adopt for long periods of time during the day in our modern world can generate retraction of the hamstrings in some people. This retraction of the muscles behind the thigh puts the pelvis into a posterior tilt at the same time as it puts the back into the poor position of losing its normal curves.

The individual assumes a poor posture, with the buttocks tucked under and the back rounded, which over time can set off vertebral pathologies. To limit this relatively frequent retraction of the hamstring muscles we recommend performing stretch exercises for the back of the thigh, such as a gentle good morning with the legs extended and gentle hip raises with extended legs. After a hamstring exercise session we recommend also performing some specific stretches.

ACTION OF THE HAMSTRINGS AND GLUTEUS MAXIMUS WHEN STRAIGHTENING THE PELVIS

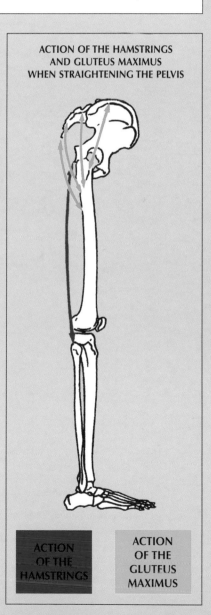

ACTION OF THE HAMSTRINGS

ACTION OF THE GLUTEUS MAXIMUS

25 GOOD MORNINGS WITH A STAFF

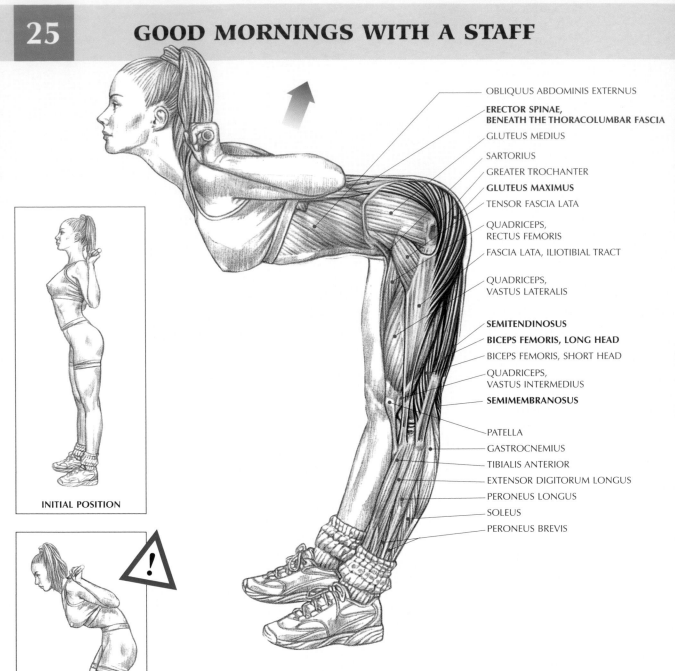

OBLIQUUS ABDOMINIS EXTERNUS

**ERECTOR SPINAE,
BENEATH THE THORACOLUMBAR FASCIA**

GLUTEUS MEDIUS

SARTORIUS

GREATER TROCHANTER

GLUTEUS MAXIMUS

TENSOR FASCIA LATA

QUADRICEPS,
RECTUS FEMORIS

FASCIA LATA, ILIOTIBIAL TRACT

QUADRICEPS,
VASTUS LATERALIS

SEMITENDINOSUS

BICEPS FEMORIS, LONG HEAD

BICEPS FEMORIS, SHORT HEAD

QUADRICEPS,
VASTUS INTERMEDIUS

SEMIMEMBRANOSUS

PATELLA

GASTROCNEMIUS

TIBIALIS ANTERIOR

EXTENSOR DIGITORUM LONGUS

PERONEUS LONGUS

SOLEUS

PERONEUS BREVIS

INITIAL POSITION

As with the good morning with a bar, it is important when executing the good morning with a staff never to round the back.

Stand, feet slightly apart, staff resting on the trapezius or a little lower on the posterior deltoids.

Inhale and flex the torso forward until horizontal, keeping the legs extended and the back good and straight; the axis of flexion passes through the coxofemoral joint. Return to the initial position, squeeze the glutes at the end of the movement, and exhale.

This exercise works the hamstrings—mainly the long head of biceps femoris, semitendinosus, and semimembranosus. The gluteus maximus and the erector muscles of the spine in the lumbar region are also worked.

Notes
- It is important to execute the movement slowly, concentrating on the feel of the muscles.
- This is an excellent warm-up and stretch for the muscles behind the thigh. Doing it regularly and integrating it between squat or hamstrings at a machine series will help avoid injuries when using heavier weights.

LYING LEG CURLS

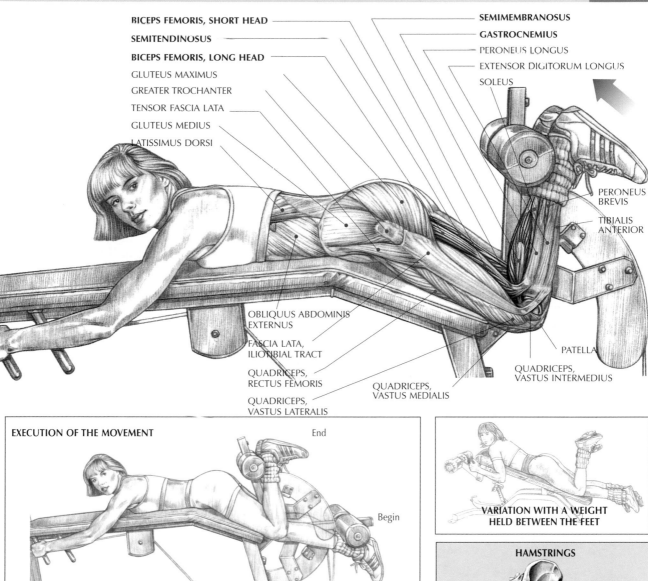

BICEPS FEMORIS, SHORT HEAD
SEMITENDINOSUS
BICEPS FEMORIS, LONG HEAD
GLUTEUS MAXIMUS
GREATER TROCHANTER
TENSOR FASCIA LATA
GLUTEUS MEDIUS
LATISSIMUS DORSI

SEMIMEMBRANOSUS
GASTROCNEMIUS
PERONEUS LONGUS
EXTENSOR DIGITORUM LONGUS
SOLEUS
PERONEUS BREVIS
TIBIALIS ANTERIOR
PATELLA
QUADRICEPS, VASTUS INTERMEDIUS

OBLIQUUS ABDOMINIS EXTERNUS
FASCIA LATA, ILIOTIBIAL TRACT
QUADRICEPS, RECTUS FEMORIS
QUADRICEPS, VASTUS LATERALIS
QUADRICEPS, VASTUS MEDIALIS

EXECUTION OF THE MOVEMENT

End

Begin

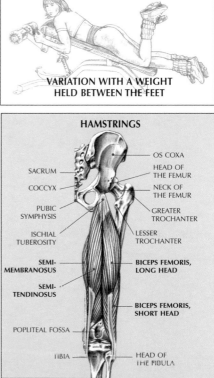

VARIATION WITH A WEIGHT HELD BETWEEN THE FEET

HAMSTRINGS

SACRUM
COCCYX
PUBIC SYMPHYSIS
ISCHIAL TUBEROSITY
SEMI-MEMBRANOSUS
SEMI-TENDINOSUS
POPLITEAL FOSSA
TIBIA

OS COXA
HEAD OF THE FEMUR
NECK OF THE FEMUR
GREATER TROCHANTER
LESSER TROCHANTER
BICEPS FEMORIS, LONG HEAD
BICEPS FEMORIS, SHORT HEAD
HEAD OF THE FIBULA

Lie flat on your belly on a machine, hands gripping the handles, legs extended, ankles engaged under the pads. Inhale and execute leg flexion with both legs simultaneously, trying to touch your buttocks with your heels. Exhale at the end of the effort. Return to the initial position with a controlled movement.

This exercise works the hamstring muscle group as well as the gastrocnemius and, deeper, the popliteus. In theory, during flexion it's possible to focus either on the semitendinosus and the semimembranosus, using internal rotation of the feet, or on the biceps femoris, long and short heads, using external rotation of the feet. In practice, however, this proves to be difficult and only focusing the work on the hamstrings or the gastrocnemius can be performed easily.

• With the feet in extension, the hamstrings are predominantly worked.
• With the feet in flexion, the gastrocnemius is predominantly worked.

Variation

It's possible to perform this movement by flexing the legs alternately.

27 STANDING LEG CURLS

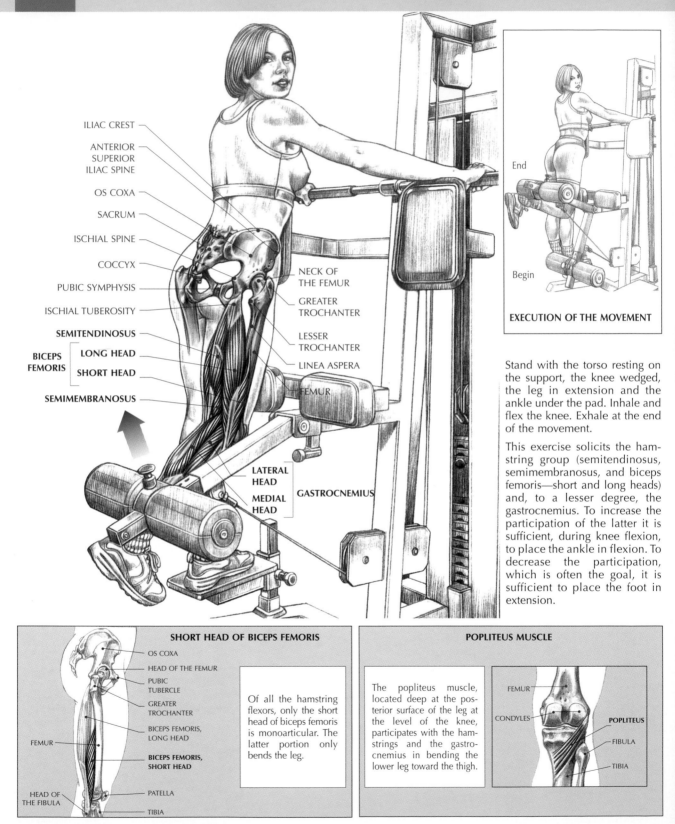

ILIAC CREST

ANTERIOR
SUPERIOR
ILIAC SPINE

OS COXA

SACRUM

ISCHIAL SPINE

COCCYX

PUBIC SYMPHYSIS

ISCHIAL TUBEROSITY

SEMITENDINOSUS

**BICEPS
FEMORIS** — **LONG HEAD**

SHORT HEAD

SEMIMEMBRANOSUS

NECK OF
THE FEMUR

GREATER
TROCHANTER

LESSER
TROCHANTER

LINEA ASPERA

FEMUR

**LATERAL
HEAD**

**MEDIAL
HEAD**

GASTROCNEMIUS

End

Begin

EXECUTION OF THE MOVEMENT

Stand with the torso resting on the support, the knee wedged, the leg in extension and the ankle under the pad. Inhale and flex the knee. Exhale at the end of the movement.

This exercise solicits the hamstring group (semitendinosus, semimembranosus, and biceps femoris—short and long heads) and, to a lesser degree, the gastrocnemius. To increase the participation of the latter it is sufficient, during knee flexion, to place the ankle in flexion. To decrease the participation, which is often the goal, it is sufficient to place the foot in extension.

SHORT HEAD OF BICEPS FEMORIS

OS COXA

HEAD OF THE FEMUR

PUBIC
TUBERCLE

GREATER
TROCHANTER

BICEPS FEMORIS,
LONG HEAD

FEMUR

**BICEPS FEMORIS,
SHORT HEAD**

HEAD OF
THE FIBULA

PATELLA

TIBIA

Of all the hamstring flexors, only the short head of biceps femoris is monoarticular. The latter portion only bends the leg.

POPLITEUS MUSCLE

The popliteus muscle, located deep at the posterior surface of the leg at the level of the knee, participates with the hamstrings and the gastrocnemius in bending the lower leg toward the thigh.

FEMUR

CONDYLES

POPLITEUS

FIBULA

TIBIA

SEATED LEG CURLS

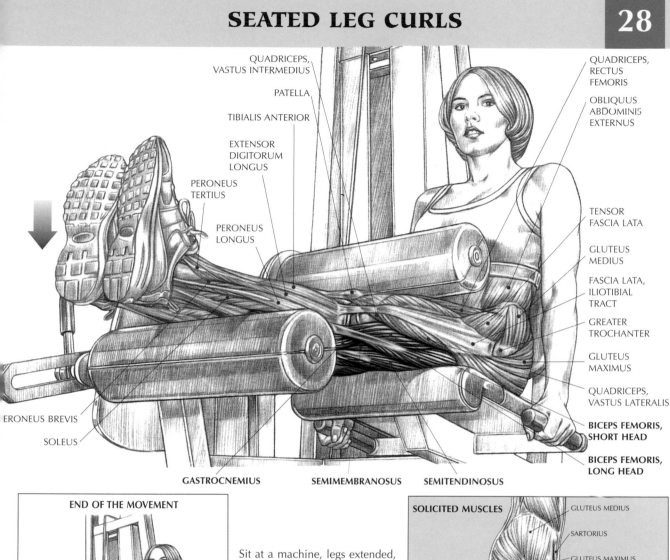

QUADRICEPS, VASTUS INTERMEDIUS

PATELLA

TIBIALIS ANTERIOR

EXTENSOR DIGITORUM LONGUS

PERONEUS TERTIUS

PERONEUS LONGUS

QUADRICEPS, RECTUS FEMORIS

OBLIQUUS ABDOMINIS EXTERNUS

TENSOR FASCIA LATA

GLUTEUS MEDIUS

FASCIA LATA, ILIOTIBIAL TRACT

GREATER TROCHANTER

GLUTEUS MAXIMUS

QUADRICEPS, VASTUS LATERALIS

BICEPS FEMORIS, SHORT HEAD

BICEPS FEMORIS, LONG HEAD

ERONEUS BREVIS

SOLEUS

GASTROCNEMIUS

SEMIMEMBRANOSUS

SEMITENDINOSUS

END OF THE MOVEMENT

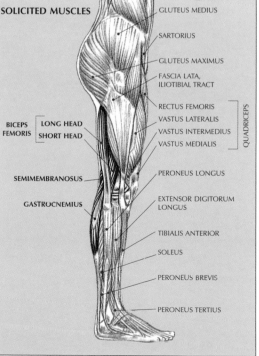

SOLICITED MUSCLES

GLUTEUS MEDIUS

SARTORIUS

GLUTEUS MAXIMUS

FASCIA LATA, ILIOTIBIAL TRACT

RECTUS FEMORIS

VASTUS LATERALIS

VASTUS INTERMEDIUS

VASTUS MEDIALIS

QUADRICEPS

BICEPS FEMORIS — LONG HEAD — SHORT HEAD

SEMIMEMBRANOSUS

GASTROCNEMIUS

PERONEUS LONGUS

EXTENSOR DIGITORUM LONGUS

TIBIALIS ANTERIOR

SOLEUS

PERONEUS BREVIS

PERONEUS TERTIUS

Sit at a machine, legs extended, ankles placed on the pad, thighs wedged, hand on the handles. Inhale and flex the legs. Exhale at the end of the movement.

This exercise solicits the hamstring group, the popliteus muscle, and to a lesser extent the gastrocnemius.

Variations

- By performing the exercise with the feet in dorsiflexion, you place part of the work on the gastrocnemius.
- By performing the exercise with the feet in extension, you focus the effort mainly onto the hamstrings.

HAMSTRINGS AT A BENCH

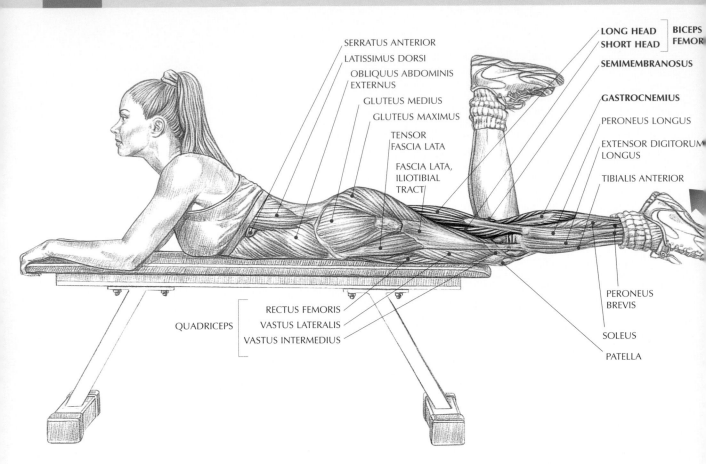

SERRATUS ANTERIOR
LATISSIMUS DORSI
OBLIQUUS ABDOMINIS EXTERNUS
GLUTEUS MEDIUS
GLUTEUS MAXIMUS
TENSOR FASCIA LATA
FASCIA LATA, ILIOTIBIAL TRACT

LONG HEAD — BICEPS
SHORT HEAD — FEMORIS
SEMIMEMBRANOSUS
GASTROCNEMIUS
PERONEUS LONGUS
EXTENSOR DIGITORUM LONGUS
TIBIALIS ANTERIOR
PERONEUS BREVIS
SOLEUS
PATELLA

QUADRICEPS
RECTUS FEMORIS
VASTUS LATERALIS
VASTUS INTERMEDIUS

Lie on your belly on a bench, head extended, knees off the bench, legs extended, feet held in extension. Simultaneously flex the legs, trying to touch the buttocks with the heels.

Return to the initial position.

This exercise works the hamstring muscle group (semimembranosus, semitendinosus, and biceps femoris) as well as the gastrocnemius muscles. This movement is performed slowly; the most important part is to concentrate on maximum contraction of the muscle at the end of the leg flexion. As with most exercises without additional weights, long series provide the best results.

Notes
- Performing thigh flexions with the feet in dorsiflexion works mainly the gastrocnemius.
- Performing thigh flexions with the feet in plantar flexion works mainly the hamstring muscles.

Variations
- For more intensity it's possible to add ankle weights.
- The load may be increased by placing a dumbbell between the ankles.

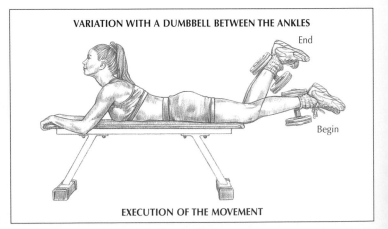

VARIATION WITH A DUMBBELL BETWEEN THE ANKLES
End
Begin
EXECUTION OF THE MOVEMENT

HAMSTRINGS ON THE FLOOR

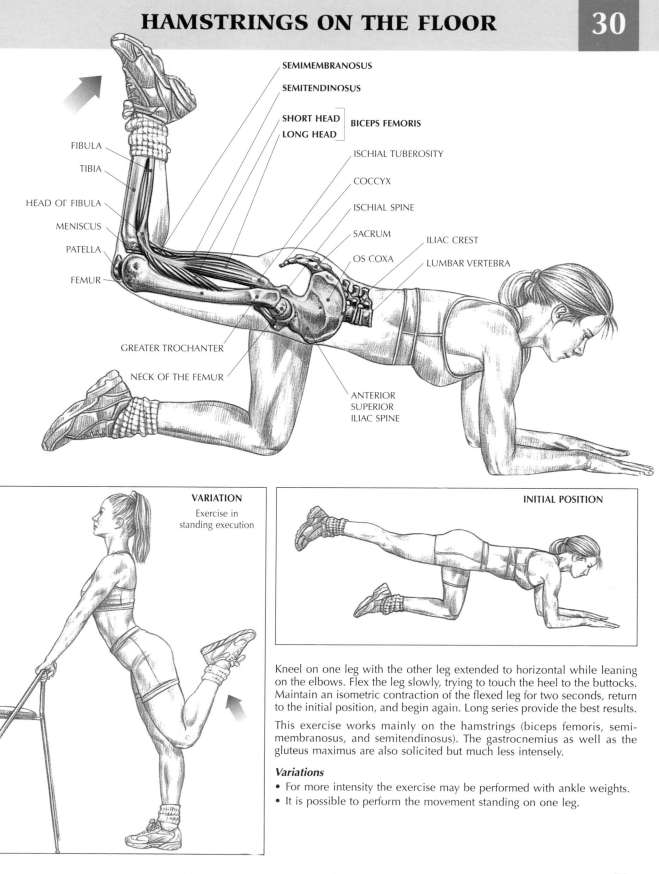

SEMIMEMBRANOSUS

SEMITENDINOSUS

SHORT HEAD
LONG HEAD **BICEPS FEMORIS**

ISCHIAL TUBEROSITY

COCCYX

ISCHIAL SPINE

SACRUM

OS COXA

ILIAC CREST

LUMBAR VERTEBRA

FIBULA

TIBIA

HEAD OF FIBULA

MENISCUS

PATELLA

FEMUR

GREATER TROCHANTER

NECK OF THE FEMUR

ANTERIOR
SUPERIOR
ILIAC SPINE

VARIATION
Exercise in
standing execution

INITIAL POSITION

Kneel on one leg with the other leg extended to horizontal while leaning
on the elbows. Flex the leg slowly, trying to touch the heel to the buttocks.
Maintain an isometric contraction of the flexed leg for two seconds, return
to the initial position, and begin again. Long series provide the best results.

This exercise works mainly on the hamstrings (biceps femoris, semimembranosus, and semitendinosus). The gastrocnemius as well as the
gluteus maximus are also solicited but much less intensely.

Variations
• For more intensity the exercise may be performed with ankle weights.
• It is possible to perform the movement standing on one leg.

31 KNEELING HAMSTRINGS

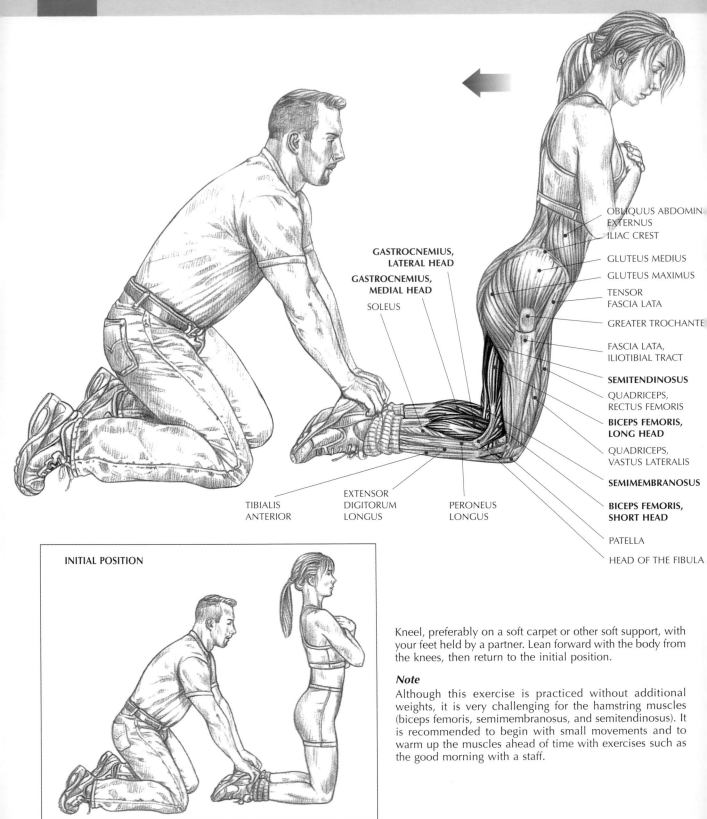

GASTROCNEMIUS,
LATERAL HEAD

GASTROCNEMIUS,
MEDIAL HEAD

SOLEUS

OBLIQUUS ABDOMIN
EXTERNUS
ILIAC CREST

GLUTEUS MEDIUS

GLUTEUS MAXIMUS

TENSOR
FASCIA LATA

GREATER TROCHANTE

FASCIA LATA,
ILIOTIBIAL TRACT

SEMITENDINOSUS

QUADRICEPS,
RECTUS FEMORIS

BICEPS FEMORIS,
LONG HEAD

QUADRICEPS,
VASTUS LATERALIS

SEMIMEMBRANOSUS

BICEPS FEMORIS,
SHORT HEAD

PATELLA

HEAD OF THE FIBULA

TIBIALIS
ANTERIOR

EXTENSOR
DIGITORUM
LONGUS

PERONEUS
LONGUS

INITIAL POSITION

Kneel, preferably on a soft carpet or other soft support, with your feet held by a partner. Lean forward with the body from the knees, then return to the initial position.

Note
Although this exercise is practiced without additional weights, it is very challenging for the hamstring muscles (biceps femoris, semimembranosus, and semitendinosus). It is recommended to begin with small movements and to warm up the muscles ahead of time with exercises such as the good morning with a staff.

STANDING CALF RAISES

EXECUTION OF THE MOVEMENT

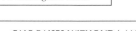

Begin   End

Variation

The execution of the exercise at an incline machine allows you to work the calves without overloading the back.

CALF RAISES WITHOUT A MACHINE

If no equipment is available to work the calves, it is possible to perform the calf raises in long series until you feel a burn. For more stability in the extensions, hold onto a chair or a stable object.

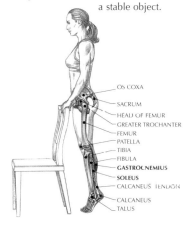

OS COXA
SACRUM
HEAD OF FEMUR
GREATER TROCHANTER
FEMUR
PATELLA
TIBIA
FIBULA
GASTROCNEMIUS
SOLEUS
CALCANEUS TENDON
CALCANEUS
TALUS

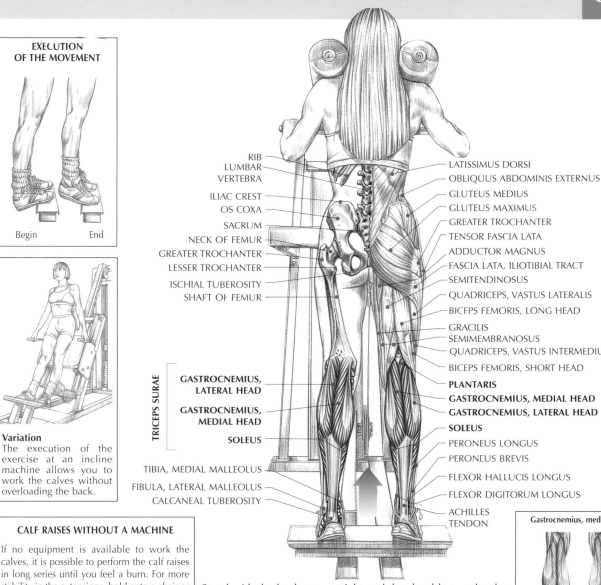

RIB
LUMBAR VERTEBRA
ILIAC CREST
OS COXA
SACRUM
NECK OF FEMUR
GREATER TROCHANTER
LESSER TROCHANTER
ISCHIAL TUBEROSITY
SHAFT OF FEMUR

LATISSIMUS DORSI
OBLIQUUS ABDOMINIS EXTERNUS
GLUTEUS MEDIUS
GLUTEUS MAXIMUS
GREATER TROCHANTER
TENSOR FASCIA LATA
ADDUCTOR MAGNUS
FASCIA LATA, ILIOTIBIAL TRACT
SEMITENDINOSUS
QUADRICEPS, VASTUS LATERALIS
BICEPS FEMORIS, LONG HEAD
GRACILIS
SEMIMEMBRANOSUS
QUADRICEPS, VASTUS INTERMEDIUS
BICEPS FEMORIS, SHORT HEAD
PLANTARIS
GASTROCNEMIUS, MEDIAL HEAD
GASTROCNEMIUS, LATERAL HEAD
SOLEUS
PERONEUS LONGUS
PERONEUS BREVIS
FLEXOR HALLUCIS LONGUS
FLEXOR DIGITORUM LONGUS
ACHILLES TENDON

TRICEPS SURAE {
GASTROCNEMIUS, LATERAL HEAD
GASTROCNEMIUS, MEDIAL HEAD
SOLEUS

TIBIA, MEDIAL MALLEOLUS
FIBULA, LATERAL MALLEOLUS
CALCANEAL TUBEROSITY

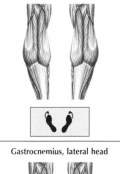

Gastrocnemius, medial head

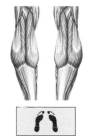

Gastrocnemius, lateral head

Stand with the back very straight and the shoulders under the padded parts of the apparatus, the balls of the feet on the platform, the ankles in easy flexion. Extend the feet (plantar flexion), always keeping the knees in extension.

This exercise solicits the triceps surae (made up of the soleus and the lateral and medial heads of the gastrocnemius). It is important to perform each repetition with a complete flexion to stretch the muscles well. In theory it is possible to localize the work onto the medial gastrocnemius (by pointing the toes outward) or onto the lateral gastrocnemius (by pointing the toes inward), but in practice this proves difficult and only dissociation between the work of the soleus and the gastrocnemius can be performed easily (by flexing the articulation at the knee to relax the gastrocnemius and put more effort on the soleus).

Variation

This movement may be performed with a frame guide with a block under the feet or with a free bar without a block for more balance but less range of motion.

DONKEY CALF RAISES

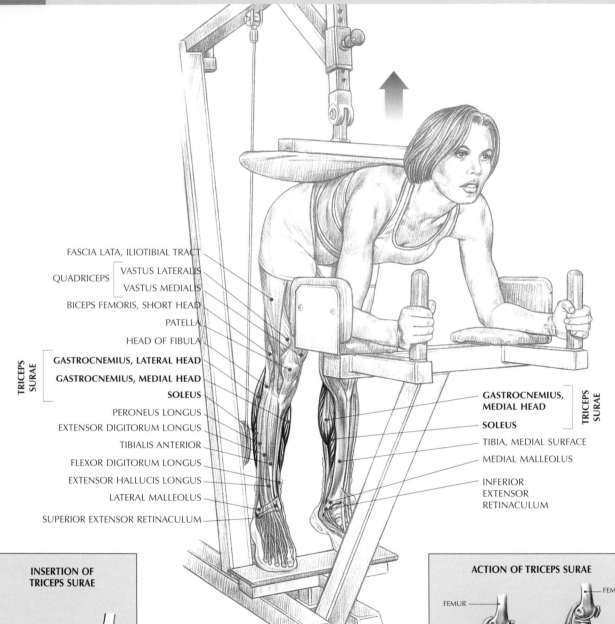

FASCIA LATA, ILIOTIBIAL TRACT

QUADRICEPS {
VASTUS LATERALIS
VASTUS MEDIALIS

BICEPS FEMORIS, SHORT HEAD

PATELLA

HEAD OF FIBULA

TRICEPS SURAE {
GASTROCNEMIUS, LATERAL HEAD
GASTROCNEMIUS, MEDIAL HEAD
SOLEUS

PERONEUS LONGUS

EXTENSOR DIGITORUM LONGUS

TIBIALIS ANTERIOR

FLEXOR DIGITORUM LONGUS

EXTENSOR HALLUCIS LONGUS

LATERAL MALLEOLUS

SUPERIOR EXTENSOR RETINACULUM

GASTROCNEMIUS, MEDIAL HEAD
SOLEUS
} TRICEPS SURAE

TIBIA, MEDIAL SURFACE

MEDIAL MALLEOLUS

INFERIOR EXTENSOR RETINACULUM

INSERTION OF TRICEPS SURAE

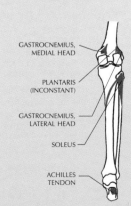

GASTROCNEMIUS, MEDIAL HEAD

PLANTARIS (INCONSTANT)

GASTROCNEMIUS, LATERAL HEAD

SOLEUS

ACHILLES TENDON

ACTION OF TRICEPS SURAE

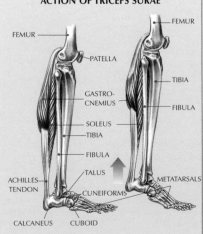

FEMUR

FEMUR

PATELLA

GASTRO-CNEMIUS

TIBIA

FIBULA

SOLEUS

TIBIA

FIBULA

TALUS

METATARSALS

ACHILLES TENDON

CUNEIFORMS

CALCANEUS

CUBOID

Place your feet on the platform in easy flexion, legs extended, torso tilted forward, forearms resting on the front support, with the padded part of the machine resting on the pelvis. Extend the feet in plantar flexion.

This exercise solicits the triceps surae, especially the gastrocnemius.

Variation

This movement can be performed with the torso flexed and a block under the feet, with the forearms resting on a support, and someone seated astride the pelvis or low back.

ONE-LEG TOE RAISES

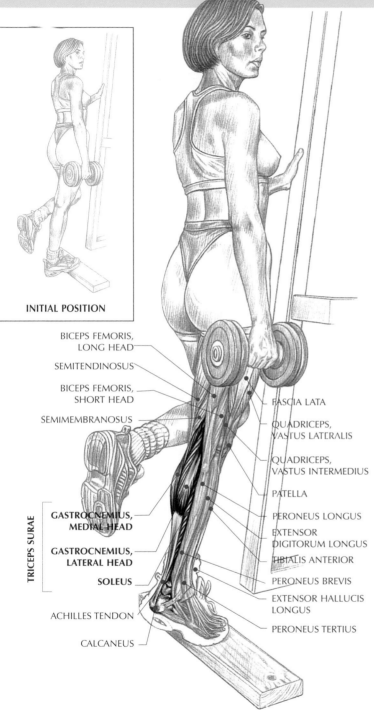

INITIAL POSITION

BICEPS FEMORIS, LONG HEAD

SEMITENDINOSUS

BICEPS FEMORIS, SHORT HEAD

SEMIMEMBRANOSUS

TRICEPS SURAE

GASTROCNEMIUS, MEDIAL HEAD

GASTROCNEMIUS, LATERAL HEAD

SOLEUS

ACHILLES TENDON

CALCANEUS

FASCIA LATA

QUADRICEPS, VASTUS LATERALIS

QUADRICEPS, VASTUS INTERMEDIUS

PATELLA

PERONEUS LONGUS

EXTENSOR DIGITORUM LONGUS

TIBIALIS ANTERIOR

PERONEUS BREVIS

EXTENSOR HALLUCIS LONGUS

PERONEUS TERTIUS

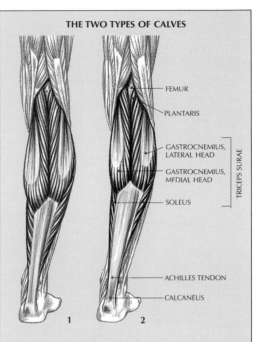

THE TWO TYPES OF CALVES

FEMUR

PLANTARIS

GASTROCNEMIUS, LATERAL HEAD

GASTROCNEMIUS, MEDIAL HEAD

SOLEUS

TRICEPS SURAE

ACHILLES TENDON

CALCANEUS

1   2

1. Long calf: gastrocnemius and soleus extend lower.
2. Short calf: gastrocnemius and soleus are very high with a long tendon.

Note

For some people the triceps surae is one of the few muscles that does not respond by an increase in volume with training. These people can only gain strength. Long calves (that is, calves where the gastrocnemius and soleus are very low) can easily develop; on the other hand, short calves will resist development.

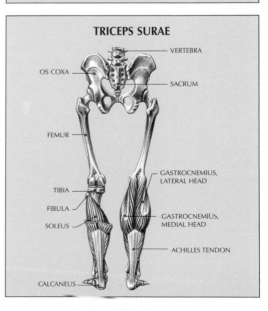

TRICEPS SURAE

VERTEBRA

OS COXA

SACRUM

FEMUR

GASTROCNEMIUS, LATERAL HEAD

TIBIA

FIBULA

GASTROCNEMIUS, MEDIAL HEAD

SOLEUS

ACHILLES TENDON

CALCANEUS

Stand on one leg with the forefoot on a block, one hand holding the dumbbell, the other gripping a support for better balance. Extend the foot (plantar flexion) keeping the articulation at the knee in extension or slightly flexed, Return to the initial position.

This exercise solicits the triceps surae (made up of the soleus and the medial and lateral heads of the gastrocnemius). It is important to flex the foot completely with each repetition to stretch the triceps surae well. Only long series until a burn sensation is felt provides good results.

35 STANDING BARBELL CALF RAISES

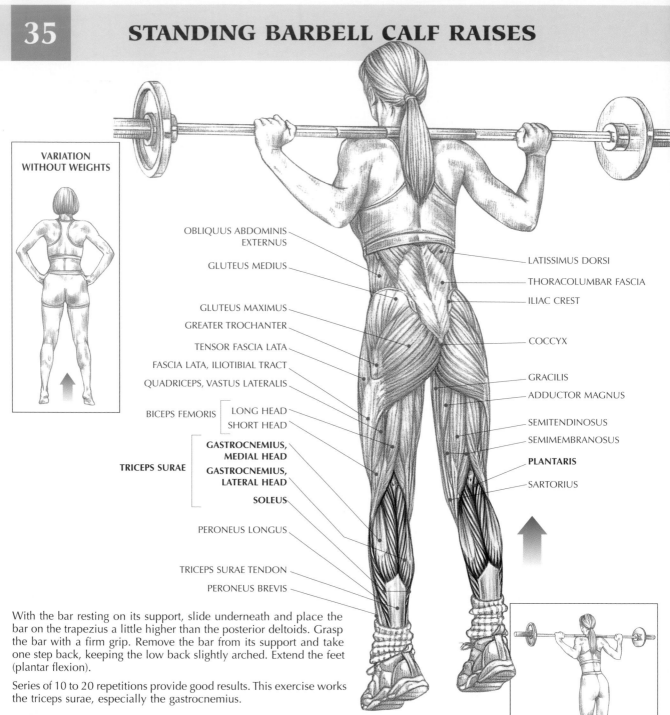

VARIATION WITHOUT WEIGHTS

OBLIQUUS ABDOMINIS EXTERNUS

GLUTEUS MEDIUS

GLUTEUS MAXIMUS

GREATER TROCHANTER

TENSOR FASCIA LATA

FASCIA LATA, ILIOTIBIAL TRACT

QUADRICEPS, VASTUS LATERALIS

BICEPS FEMORIS — LONG HEAD / SHORT HEAD

TRICEPS SURAE — **GASTROCNEMIUS, MEDIAL HEAD** / **GASTROCNEMIUS, LATERAL HEAD** / **SOLEUS**

PERONEUS LONGUS

TRICEPS SURAE TENDON

PERONEUS BREVIS

LATISSIMUS DORSI

THORACOLUMBAR FASCIA

ILIAC CREST

COCCYX

GRACILIS

ADDUCTOR MAGNUS

SEMITENDINOSUS

SEMIMEMBRANOSUS

PLANTARIS

SARTORIUS

With the bar resting on its support, slide underneath and place the bar on the trapezius a little higher than the posterior deltoids. Grasp the bar with a firm grip. Remove the bar from its support and take one step back, keeping the low back slightly arched. Extend the feet (plantar flexion).

Series of 10 to 20 repetitions provide good results. This exercise works the triceps surae, especially the gastrocnemius.

Variation

Without equipment, it is possible to perform feet extensions in long series until you feel a burn. To feel the calves working properly, it is possible to move on to an exercise with weights immediately after a long series without equipment.

Example

20 repetitions of calf raises at a machine or with a bar followed by 50 feet extensions.

INITIAL POSITION

> **Note**
> As the triceps surae is an extremely powerful and resistant muscle, which by itself lifts the weight of the body thousands of times a day when you walk, do not hesitate to work it with heavy weight.

SEATED BARBELL CALF RAISES

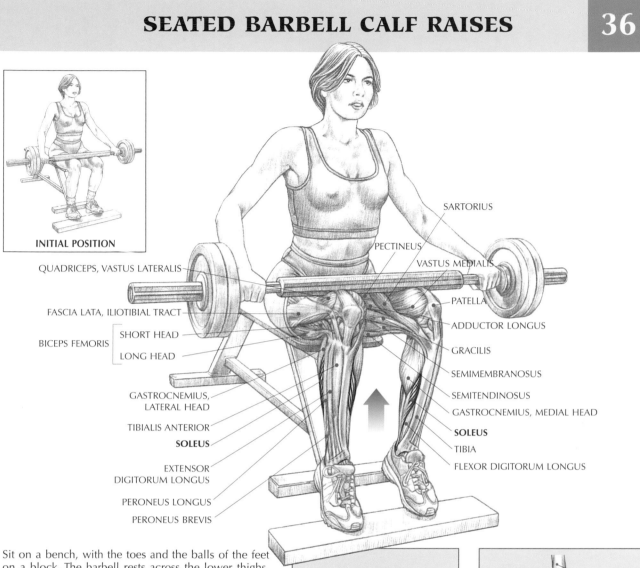

INITIAL POSITION

QUADRICEPS, VASTUS LATERALIS

FASCIA LATA, ILIOTIBIAL TRACT

BICEPS FEMORIS
- SHORT HEAD
- LONG HEAD

GASTROCNEMIUS, LATERAL HEAD

TIBIALIS ANTERIOR

SOLEUS

EXTENSOR DIGITORUM LONGUS

PERONEUS LONGUS

PERONEUS BREVIS

SARTORIUS

PECTINEUS

VASTUS MEDIALIS

PATELLA

ADDUCTOR LONGUS

GRACILIS

SEMIMEMBRANOSUS

SEMITENDINOSUS

GASTROCNEMIUS, MEDIAL HEAD

SOLEUS

TIBIA

FLEXOR DIGITORUM LONGUS

Sit on a bench, with the toes and the balls of the feet on a block. The barbell rests across the lower thighs. Perform extension of the feet (plantar flexion).

Note

We recommend placing a rubber pad on the bar or, failing that, a folded towel on the thighs or wrapped around the bar to make the exercise more comfortable.

This exercise solicits mainly the soleus. This muscle makes up part of the triceps surae and inserts superiorly below the articulation at the knee onto the tibia and the fibula. It is attached below onto the calcaneus via the Achilles tendon, and its function is to extend the ankles. Unlike the soleus press, which allows for working with heavy weights, this exercise cannot be performed with very heavy weight. For the best results it is therefore recommended to work in series of 15 to 20 repetitions.

Variation

It is possible to perform this movement without additional weight on a chair or bench. In this case you will have to execute very long series until you feel a burn.

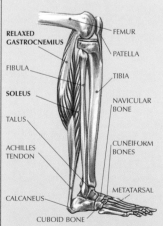

RELAXED GASTROCNEMIUS

FEMUR

PATELLA

FIBULA

TIBIA

SOLEUS

NAVICULAR BONE

TALUS

CUNEIFORM BONES

ACHILLES TENDON

CALCANEUS

METATARSAL

CUBOID BONE

1. When the knees are flexed, the gastrocnemius muscles (which attach superior to the articulation at the knee) are relaxed. In this position they only participate weakly with foot extension, with most of the work being performed by the soleus muscle.

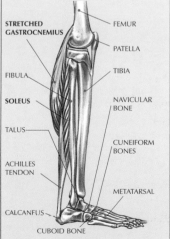

STRETCHED GASTROCNEMIUS

FEMUR

PATELLA

FIBULA

TIBIA

SOLEUS

NAVICULAR BONE

TALUS

CUNEIFORM BONES

ACHILLES TENDON

METATARSAL

CALCANEUS

CUBOID BONE

2. When the articulation of the knee is in extension, the gastrocnemius muscles are stretched. In this position they actively participate in extension of the feet and complement the action of the soleus.

SEATED CALF RAISES

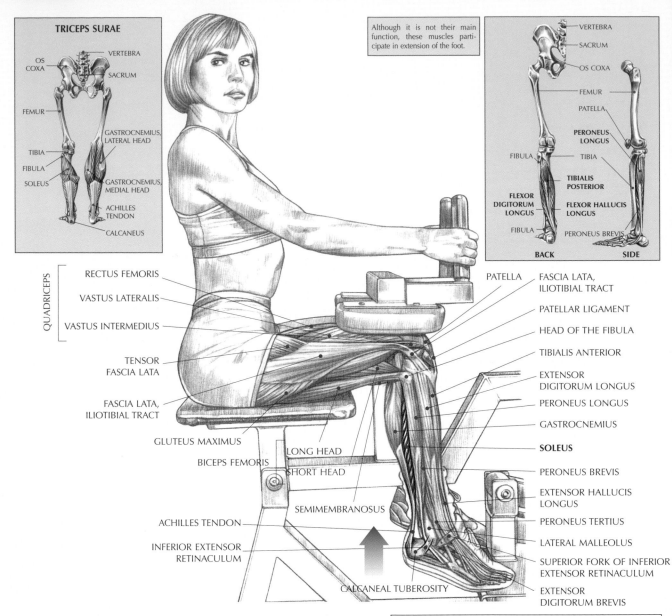

TRICEPS SURAE

OS COXA
VERTEBRA
SACRUM
FEMUR
TIBIA
FIBULA
SOLEUS
GASTROCNEMIUS, LATERAL HEAD
GASTROCNEMIUS, MEDIAL HEAD
ACHILLES TENDON
CALCANEUS

Although it is not their main function, these muscles participate in extension of the foot.

VERTEBRA
SACRUM
OS COXA
FEMUR
PATELLA
PERONEUS LONGUS
FIBULA
TIBIA
TIBIALIS POSTERIOR
FLEXOR DIGITORUM LONGUS
FLEXOR HALLUCIS LONGUS
FIBULA
PERONEUS BREVIS
BACK   **SIDE**

QUADRICEPS
RECTUS FEMORIS
VASTUS LATERALIS
VASTUS INTERMEDIUS
TENSOR FASCIA LATA
FASCIA LATA, ILIOTIBIAL TRACT
GLUTEUS MAXIMUS
BICEPS FEMORIS
LONG HEAD
SHORT HEAD
SEMIMEMBRANOSUS
ACHILLES TENDON
INFERIOR EXTENSOR RETINACULUM
CALCANEAL TUBEROSITY

PATELLA
FASCIA LATA, ILIOTIBIAL TRACT
PATELLAR LIGAMENT
HEAD OF THE FIBULA
TIBIALIS ANTERIOR
EXTENSOR DIGITORUM LONGUS
PERONEUS LONGUS
GASTROCNEMIUS
SOLEUS
PERONEUS BREVIS
EXTENSOR HALLUCIS LONGUS
PERONEUS TERTIUS
LATERAL MALLEOLUS
SUPERIOR FORK OF INFERIOR EXTENSOR RETINACULUM
EXTENSOR DIGITORUM BREVIS

Sit at a machine, with the restraint pads across the lower thighs, the anterior part of the feet on the pedestal, the ankles in easy flexion. Extend the feet (plantar flexion).

This exercise essentially solicits the soleus muscle (this muscle inserts high up below the articulation at the knee onto the tibia and fibula and is attached to the calcaneus by the Achilles tendon; its function is to extend the ankles). The flexed position of the knees relaxes the gastrocnemius, which attach superior to the articulation at the knee and inferiorly to the Achilles tendon, so that they only weakly participate in foot extension.

Variation

The movement can be performed seated at a bench with a wedge under the feet and a bar placed on the lower part of the thighs. In this case a rubber pad should be placed on the bar (or a rolled towel on the thighs) to make the exercise more comfortable.

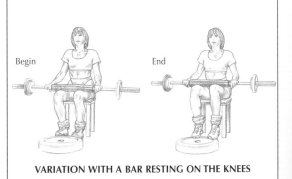

Begin   End

VARIATION WITH A BAR RESTING ON THE KNEES

ABDOMINALS

III

1. CRUNCHES
2. CRUNCHES WITH FEET ON THE FLOOR
3. CRUNCHES AT A MACHINE
4. TORSO RAISES OFF THE FLOOR
5. HALF CRUNCHES
6. CRUNCHES WITH FEET RAISED
7. LEG EXTENSIONS ON THE FLOOR
8. LEG EXTENSIONS ON THE FLOOR WITH FEET RAISED
9. CRUNCHES ON A WALL BAR
10. CRUNCHES ON A BENCH
11. CRUNCHES ON AN INCLINE BENCH
12. CRUNCHES ON AN INCLINE BOARD
13. SUSPENDED CRUNCHES AT A BENCH
14. LEG RAISES IN AN ABDOMINAL CHAIR
15. LEG RAISES FROM A FIXED BAR
16. LEG RAISES ON AN INCLINE BOARD WITH CRUNCHES
17. PELVIC LIFTS OFF THE FLOOR
18. PELVIC ROTATIONS ON THE FLOOR
19. OBLIQUE CRUNCHES WITH FEET ON THE FLOOR
20. CYCLING (OR ALTERNATING OBLIQUES) ON THE FLOOR
21. SIDELYING TORSO FLEXIONS
22. HIGH PULLEY CRUNCHES
23. MACHINE CRUNCHES
24. LATERAL TORSO FLEXIONS ON A BENCH
25. OBLIQUES AT A ROCKING MACHINE
26. LATERAL TORSO FLEXIONS AT A LOW PULLEY
27. OBLIQUES AT A HIGH PULLEY
28. LATERAL TORSO FLEXIONS WITH DUMBBELLS
29. BROOMSTICK TWISTS
30. SEATED BROOMSTICK TWISTS
31. SEATED TORSO ROTATIONS AT A TWIST MACHINE
32. STANDING TORSO ROTATIONS AT A TWIST MACHINE
33. SEATED TUMMY SUCKS
34. ABDOMINALS IN HORIZONTAL STABILIZATION

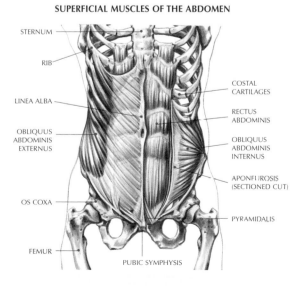

SUPERFICIAL MUSCLES OF THE ABDOMEN

STERNUM
RIB
LINEA ALBA
OBLIQUUS ABDOMINIS EXTERNUS
OS COXA
FEMUR
PUBIC SYMPHYSIS
COSTAL CARTILAGES
RECTUS ABDOMINIS
OBLIQUUS ABDOMINIS INTERNUS
APONEUROSIS (SECTIONED CUT)
PYRAMIDALIS

DEEP MUSCLES OF THE ABDOMEN

STERNUM
RIB
XIPHOID PROCESS
COSTAL CARTILAGES
VERTEBRA
OS COXA
SACRUM
FEMUR
PUBIC SYMPHYSIS
LINEA ALBA
TRANSVERSUS ABDOMINIS
APONEUROSIS
RECTUS ABDOMINIS (CUT)
INGUINAL LIGAMENT

WARNING

Unlike the other movements in weight lifting, the exercises for the abdominal muscles, and especially those for the rectus abdominis, must absolutely be worked with a rounded back.

With rounded-back exercises on the floor, such as crunches, the mechanical constraints on the articulations of the vertebrae are not the same as in the squat, the raise from the floor, or other standing exercises.

In fact, if during the squat, the good morning, or other exercises with weights, the vertebral column is not arched at the lumbar level, the significant vertical pressure associated with rounding of the spine sends the nucleus pulposus of the intervertebral posterior, which can compress the neural elements and provoke sciatica because of disc herniation.

On the contrary, if while performing specific abdominal exercises we forget to round the back with an intense contraction of the rectus and oblique abdominals, the powerful hip flexors, which are the psoas major, tend to accentuate the lumbar arch, sending the intervertebral discs that are not stabilized by vertical pressure forward. There then follows excessive pressure at the back of the lumbar vertebrae, which can lead to back pain or more seriously to articular deterioration by compression and shearing.

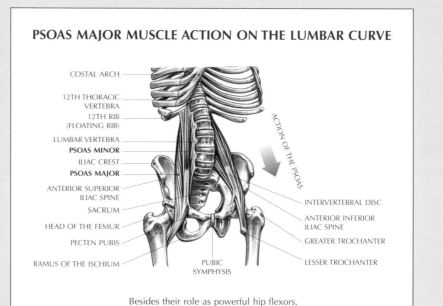

PSOAS MAJOR MUSCLE ACTION ON THE LUMBAR CURVE

COSTAL ARCH

12TH THORACIC VERTEBRA

12TH RIB (FLOATING RIB)

LUMBAR VERTEBRA

PSOAS MINOR

ILIAC CREST

PSOAS MAJOR

ANTERIOR SUPERIOR ILIAC SPINE

SACRUM

HEAD OF THE FEMUR

PECTEN PUBIS

RAMUS OF THE ISCHIUM

ACTION OF THE PSOAS

INTERVERTEBRAL DISC

ANTERIOR INFERIOR ILIAC SPINE

GREATER TROCHANTER

LESSER TROCHANTER

PUBIC SYMPHYSIS

Besides their role as powerful hip flexors,
the psoas muscles pull the lumbar spine into lordosis, increasing the arch.

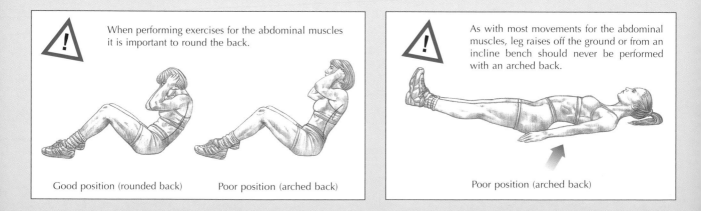

When performing exercises for the abdominal muscles it is important to round the back.

Good position (rounded back)   Poor position (arched back)

As with most movements for the abdominal muscles, leg raises off the ground or from an incline bench should never be performed with an arched back.

Poor position (arched back)

CRUNCHES

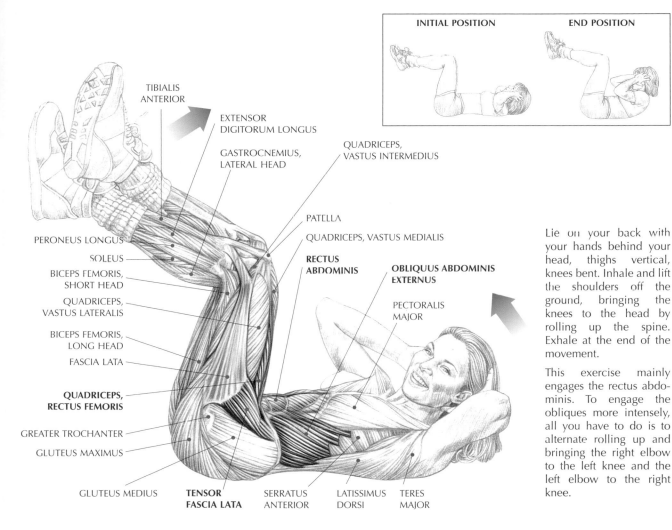

INITIAL POSITION

END POSITION

TIBIALIS
ANTERIOR

EXTENSOR
DIGITORUM LONGUS

GASTROCNEMIUS,
LATERAL HEAD

QUADRICEPS,
VASTUS INTERMEDIUS

PATELLA

QUADRICEPS, VASTUS MEDIALIS

**RECTUS
ABDOMINIS**

**OBLIQUUS ABDOMINIS
EXTERNUS**

PECTORALIS
MAJOR

PERONEUS LONGUS

SOLEUS

BICEPS FEMORIS,
SHORT HEAD

QUADRICEPS,
VASTUS LATERALIS

BICEPS FEMORIS,
LONG HEAD

FASCIA LATA

**QUADRICEPS,
RECTUS FEMORIS**

GREATER TROCHANTER

GLUTEUS MAXIMUS

GLUTEUS MEDIUS

**TENSOR
FASCIA LATA**

SERRATUS
ANTERIOR

LATISSIMUS
DORSI

TERES
MAJOR

Lie on your back with your hands behind your head, thighs vertical, knees bent. Inhale and lift the shoulders off the ground, bringing the knees to the head by rolling up the spine. Exhale at the end of the movement.

This exercise mainly engages the rectus abdominis. To engage the obliques more intensely, all you have to do is to alternate rolling up and bringing the right elbow to the left knee and the left elbow to the right knee.

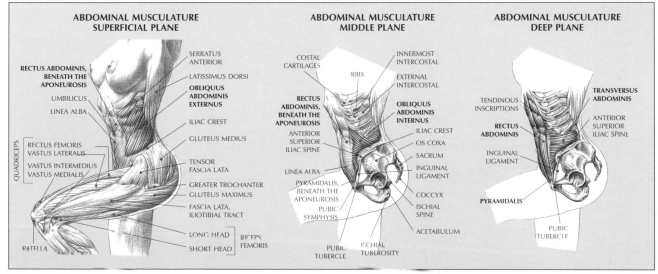

**ABDOMINAL MUSCULATURE
SUPERFICIAL PLANE**

SERRATUS
ANTERIOR

LATISSIMUS DORSI

**OBLIQUUS
ABDOMINIS
EXTERNUS**

ILIAC CREST

GLUTEUS MEDIUS

TENSOR
FASCIA LATA

GREATER TROCHANTER

GLUTEUS MAXIMUS

FASCIA LATA,
ILIOTIBIAL TRACT

LONG HEAD

SHORT HEAD

BICEPS
FEMORIS

**RECTUS ABDOMINIS,
BENEATH THE
APONEUROSIS**

UMBILICUS

LINEA ALBA

RECTUS FEMORIS
VASTUS LATERALIS

VASTUS INTERMEDIUS
VASTUS MEDIALIS

QUADRICEPS

PATELLA

**ABDOMINAL MUSCULATURE
MIDDLE PLANE**

COSTAL
CARTILAGES

RIBS

INNERMOST
INTERCOSTAL

EXTERNAL
INTERCOSTAL

**RECTUS
ABDOMINIS,
BENEATH THE
APONEUROSIS**

ANTERIOR
SUPERIOR
ILIAC SPINE

LINEA ALBA

PYRAMIDALIS,
BENEATH THE
APONEUROSIS

PUBIC
SYMPHYSIS

PUBIC
TUBERCLE

ISCHIAL
TUBEROSITY

**OBLIQUUS
ABDOMINIS
INTERNUS**

ILIAC CREST

OS COXA

SACRUM

INGUINAL
LIGAMENT

COCCYX

ISCHIAL
SPINE

ACETABULUM

**ABDOMINAL MUSCULATURE
DEEP PLANE**

TENDINOUS
INSCRIPTIONS

**RECTUS
ABDOMINIS**

INGUINAL
LIGAMENT

PYRAMIDALIS

**TRANSVERSUS
ABDOMINIS**

ANTERIOR
SUPERIOR
ILIAC SPINE

PUBIC
TUBERCLE

2

CRUNCHES WITH FEET
ON THE FLOOR

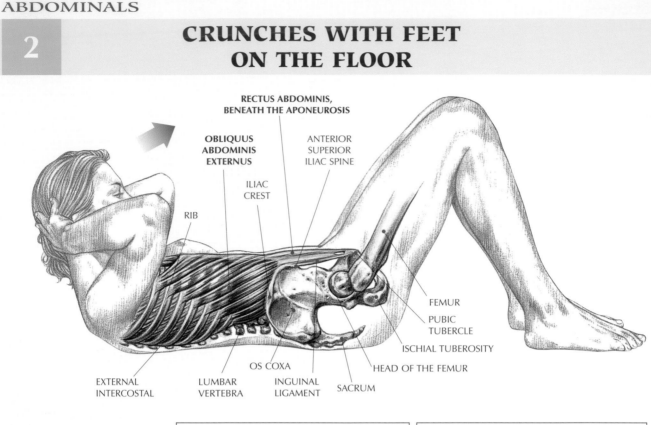

RECTUS ABDOMINIS,
BENEATH THE APONEUROSIS

OBLIQUUS
ABDOMINIS
EXTERNUS

ANTERIOR
SUPERIOR
ILIAC SPINE

ILIAC
CREST

RIB

FEMUR

PUBIC
TUBERCLE

ISCHIAL TUBEROSITY

HEAD OF THE FEMUR

EXTERNAL
INTERCOSTAL

LUMBAR
VERTEBRA

OS COXA

INGUINAL
LIGAMENT

SACRUM

Lie on the back with the hands behind the head, knees bent, feet on the floor. Inhale and lift the shoulders off the floor by rounding the back. Exhale at the end of the movement.

This exercise works the rectus muscles of the abdomen, mainly the portion below the umbilicus and to a lesser degree the oblique muscles of the abdomen.

INITIAL POSITION

END POSITION

The crunch with the feet on the floor is an excellent initiation into working the abdominal muscles. It can be performed without risk for those suffering from back pain. It is also an excellent movement for restoring abdominal tone after childbirth. Long, slow series provide the best results.

Note

As with all exercises that work the abdominal muscles, it is recommended to look toward your abdomen by bringing the chin to the chest; this position generally engages the rectus abdominis muscle in a slight reflex contraction.

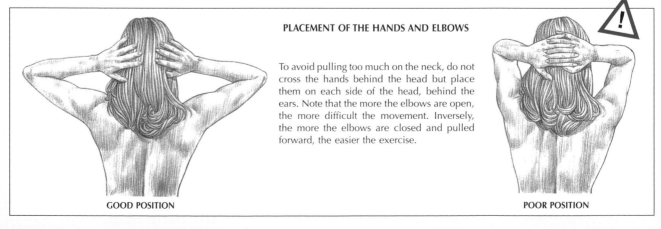

PLACEMENT OF THE HANDS AND ELBOWS

To avoid pulling too much on the neck, do not cross the hands behind the head but place them on each side of the head, behind the ears. Note that the more the elbows are open, the more difficult the movement. Inversely, the more the elbows are closed and pulled forward, the easier the exercise.

GOOD POSITION

POOR POSITION

CRUNCHES AT A MACHINE

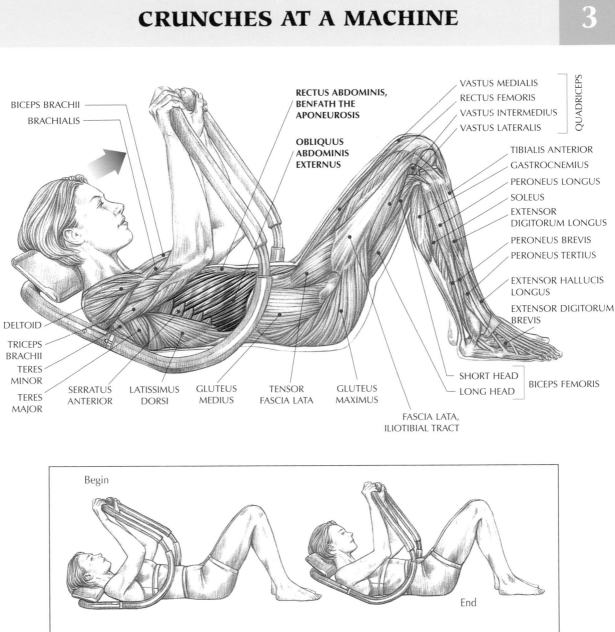

BICEPS BRACHII

BRACHIALIS

RECTUS ABDOMINIS,
BENFATH THE
APONEUROSIS

OBLIQUUS
ABDOMINIS
EXTERNUS

VASTUS MEDIALIS

RECTUS FEMORIS

VASTUS INTERMEDIUS

VASTUS LATERALIS

QUADRICEPS

TIBIALIS ANTERIOR

GASTROCNEMIUS

PERONEUS LONGUS

SOLEUS

EXTENSOR
DIGITORUM LONGUS

PERONEUS BREVIS

PERONEUS TERTIUS

EXTENSOR HALLUCIS
LONGUS

EXTENSOR DIGITORUM
BREVIS

DELTOID

TRICEPS
BRACHII

TERES
MINOR

TERES
MAJOR

SERRATUS
ANTERIOR

LATISSIMUS
DORSI

GLUTEUS
MEDIUS

TENSOR
FASCIA LATA

GLUTEUS
MAXIMUS

FASCIA LATA,
ILIOTIBIAL TRACT

SHORT HEAD

LONG HEAD

BICEPS FEMORIS

Begin

End

EXECUTION OF THE MOVEMENT

Lie on your back with your head resting on the headrest, hands on the high part of the handles, knees flexed, feet on the ground. Inhale and raise the torso as high as possible while rounding the back, keeping the head on the headrest and the low back tight against the ground. Exhale at the end of the movement.

This exercise works mainly on the superior part of the rectus muscles of the abdomen. The internal and external obliques are also worked. Long series of ten to twenty repetitions provide very good results.

Note
This is one of the rare exercises that allows the beginner to feel all the abdominal muscles working.

Variation
The lower the hands are placed on the handles, the more effort the exercise will take.

ABDOMINALS

4 TORSO RAISES OFF THE FLOOR

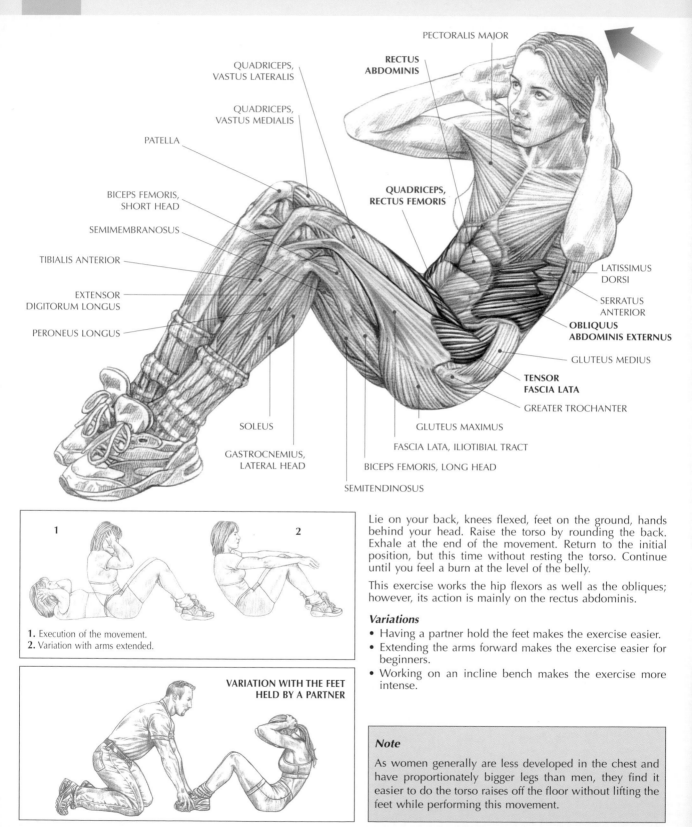

PECTORALIS MAJOR

RECTUS ABDOMINIS

QUADRICEPS, VASTUS LATERALIS

QUADRICEPS, VASTUS MEDIALIS

PATELLA

BICEPS FEMORIS, SHORT HEAD

SEMIMEMBRANOSUS

TIBIALIS ANTERIOR

EXTENSOR DIGITORUM LONGUS

PERONEUS LONGUS

QUADRICEPS, RECTUS FEMORIS

LATISSIMUS DORSI

SERRATUS ANTERIOR

OBLIQUUS ABDOMINIS EXTERNUS

GLUTEUS MEDIUS

TENSOR FASCIA LATA

GREATER TROCHANTER

SOLEUS

GASTROCNEMIUS, LATERAL HEAD

GLUTEUS MAXIMUS

FASCIA LATA, ILIOTIBIAL TRACT

BICEPS FEMORIS, LONG HEAD

SEMITENDINOSUS

1. Execution of the movement.
2. Variation with arms extended.

VARIATION WITH THE FEET HELD BY A PARTNER

Lie on your back, knees flexed, feet on the ground, hands behind your head. Raise the torso by rounding the back. Exhale at the end of the movement. Return to the initial position, but this time without resting the torso. Continue until you feel a burn at the level of the belly.

This exercise works the hip flexors as well as the obliques; however, its action is mainly on the rectus abdominis.

Variations
- Having a partner hold the feet makes the exercise easier.
- Extending the arms forward makes the exercise easier for beginners.
- Working on an incline bench makes the exercise more intense.

Note
As women generally are less developed in the chest and have proportionately bigger legs than men, they find it easier to do the torso raises off the floor without lifting the feet while performing this movement.

92

MUSCLES SOLICITED DURING THE CRUNCH

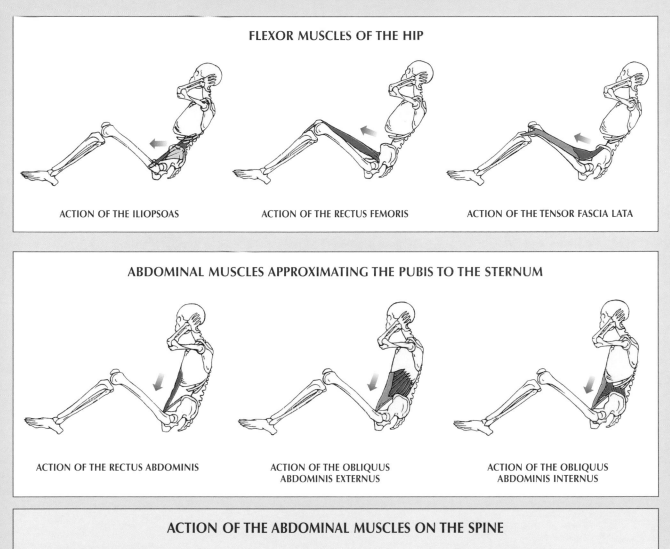

FLEXOR MUSCLES OF THE HIP

ACTION OF THE ILIOPSOAS

ACTION OF THE RECTUS FEMORIS

ACTION OF THE TENSOR FASCIA LATA

ABDOMINAL MUSCLES APPROXIMATING THE PUBIS TO THE STERNUM

ACTION OF THE RECTUS ABDOMINIS

ACTION OF THE OBLIQUUS ABDOMINIS EXTERNUS

ACTION OF THE OBLIQUUS ABDOMINIS INTERNUS

ACTION OF THE ABDOMINAL MUSCLES ON THE SPINE

MUSCLE CATEGORIES	MAIN MUSCLES	ACCESSORY MUSCLES
FLEXORS	RECTUS ABDOMINUS	EXTERNAL OBLIQUES INTERNAL OBLIQUES ILIOPSOAS
LATERAL FLEXORS	EXTERNAL OBLIQUES INTERNAL OBLIQUES QUADRATUS LUMBORUM SPINALS	RECTUS ABDOMINIS
ROTATORS	EXTERNAL OBLIQUES INTERNAL OBLIQUES SPINALS	
EXTENSORS	SPINALS	LATISSIMUS DORSI

5

HALF CRUNCHES

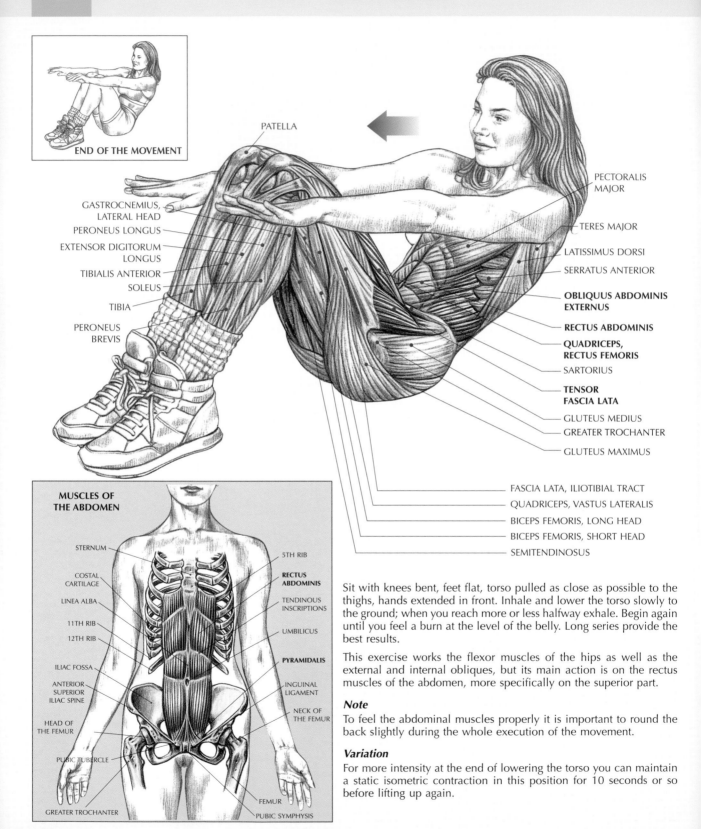

END OF THE MOVEMENT

PATELLA

GASTROCNEMIUS, LATERAL HEAD
PERONEUS LONGUS
EXTENSOR DIGITORUM LONGUS
TIBIALIS ANTERIOR
SOLEUS
TIBIA
PERONEUS BREVIS

PECTORALIS MAJOR
TERES MAJOR
LATISSIMUS DORSI
SERRATUS ANTERIOR
OBLIQUUS ABDOMINIS EXTERNUS
RECTUS ABDOMINIS
QUADRICEPS, RECTUS FEMORIS
SARTORIUS
TENSOR FASCIA LATA
GLUTEUS MEDIUS
GREATER TROCHANTER
GLUTEUS MAXIMUS

FASCIA LATA, ILIOTIBIAL TRACT
QUADRICEPS, VASTUS LATERALIS
BICEPS FEMORIS, LONG HEAD
BICEPS FEMORIS, SHORT HEAD
SEMITENDINOSUS

MUSCLES OF THE ABDOMEN

STERNUM
COSTAL CARTILAGE
LINEA ALBA
11TH RIB
12TH RIB
ILIAC FOSSA
ANTERIOR SUPERIOR ILIAC SPINE
HEAD OF THE FEMUR
PUBIC TUBERCLE
GREATER TROCHANTER

5TH RIB
RECTUS ABDOMINIS
TENDINOUS INSCRIPTIONS
UMBILICUS
PYRAMIDALIS
INGUINAL LIGAMENT
NECK OF THE FEMUR
FEMUR
PUBIC SYMPHYSIS

Sit with knees bent, feet flat, torso pulled as close as possible to the thighs, hands extended in front. Inhale and lower the torso slowly to the ground; when you reach more or less halfway exhale. Begin again until you feel a burn at the level of the belly. Long series provide the best results.

This exercise works the flexor muscles of the hips as well as the external and internal obliques, but its main action is on the rectus muscles of the abdomen, more specifically on the superior part.

Note
To feel the abdominal muscles properly it is important to round the back slightly during the whole execution of the movement.

Variation
For more intensity at the end of lowering the torso you can maintain a static isometric contraction in this position for 10 seconds or so before lifting up again.

CRUNCHES WITH FEET RAISED

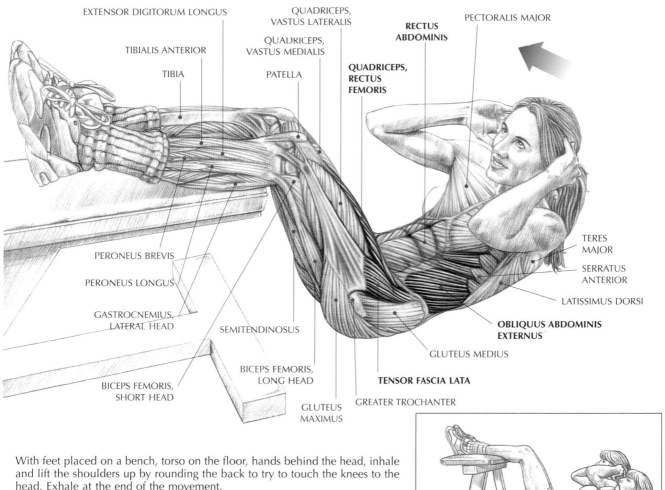

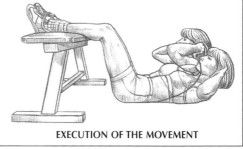

With feet placed on a bench, torso on the floor, hands behind the head, inhale and lift the shoulders up by rounding the back to try to touch the knees to the head. Exhale at the end of the movement.

This exercise focuses the effort onto the rectus abdominis, more intensely on the part below the umbilicus. Note that moving the torso away from the bench increases the mobility of the pelvis, which allows the torso to raise by flexing at the hips by contracting the iliopsoas, tensor fascia lata, and rectus femoris muscles.

EXECUTION OF THE MOVEMENT

HOW TO WORK THE ABDOMINALS AFTER CHILDBIRTH

As the muscles of the abdomen have been distended after pregnancy, it is important to do exercises that tone and shorten them. Toward this end, crunches or spinal roll-ups worked in small amplitude, keeping the back always rounded, are strongly recommended.

Warning

To avoid exaggerating the stretch of the abdominal muscles, all exercises of large amplitude (such as leg raises, torso raises, or leg extensions on the floor) should be avoided until the abdominal muscles have been toned.

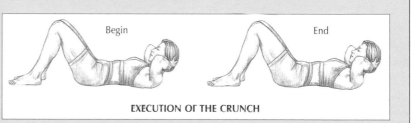

Begin

End

EXECUTION OF THE CRUNCH

7 LEG EXTENSIONS ON THE FLOOR

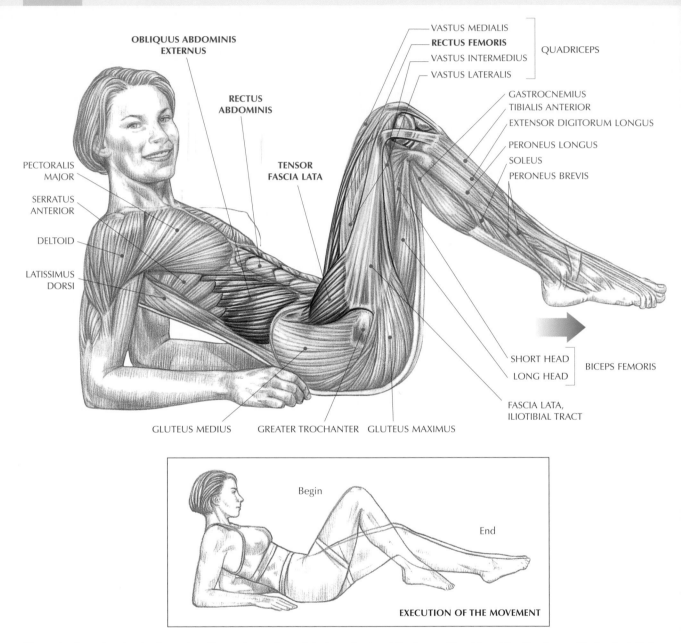

OBLIQUUS ABDOMINIS
EXTERNUS

VASTUS MEDIALIS
RECTUS FEMORIS
VASTUS INTERMEDIUS
VASTUS LATERALIS
QUADRICEPS

RECTUS
ABDOMINIS

GASTROCNEMIUS
TIBIALIS ANTERIOR
EXTENSOR DIGITORUM LONGUS

PERONEUS LONGUS
SOLEUS
PERONEUS BREVIS

TENSOR
FASCIA LATA

PECTORALIS
MAJOR

SERRATUS
ANTERIOR

DELTOID

LATISSIMUS
DORSI

SHORT HEAD
LONG HEAD
BICEPS FEMORIS

FASCIA LATA,
ILIOTIBIAL TRACT

GLUTEUS MEDIUS   GREATER TROCHANTER   GLUTEUS MAXIMUS

Begin

End

EXECUTION OF THE MOVEMENT

Sit on the floor, leaning back on the elbows, knees bent. Inhale and extend the legs without touching the floor with the feet. Return to the initial position while contracting the abdominal muscles to the maximum and exhale. This exercise should always be performed slowly without jerking.

To feel the abdominal muscles working and to avoid contractures in the lumbar region, gently round the back during the performance. As with all abdominal movements, long series provide the best results.

Leg extensions on the floor mainly solicit the rectus abdominis muscles of the abdomen, the external and internal obliques, and the flexor muscle group of the hip (the tensor fascia lata, rectus femoris, and iliopsoas).

Note
When the feet are farther away from the body, the ventral stretch is intense. For this reason women who have recently given birth need to avoid this exercise so as not to exaggerate the pull on the abdominal muscles.

LEG EXTENSIONS ON THE FLOOR
WITH FEET RAISED

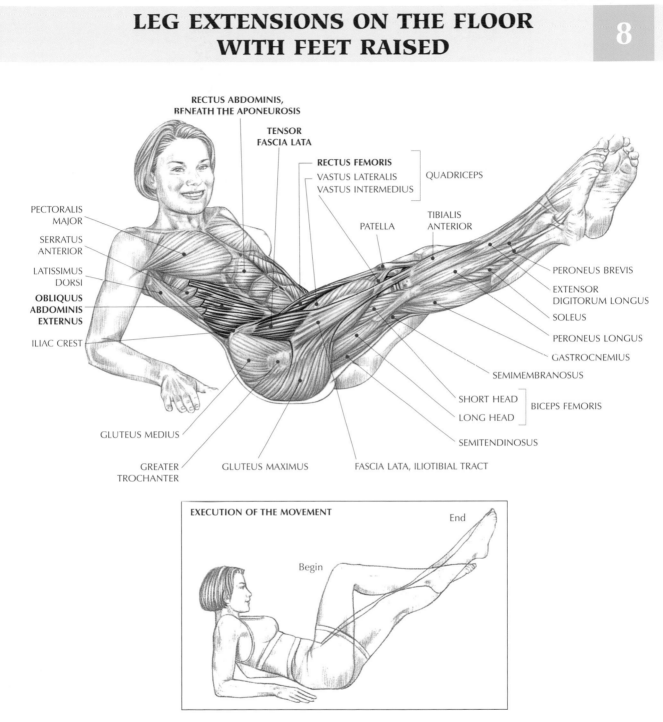

RECTUS ABDOMINIS,
BENEATH THE APONEUROSIS

TENSOR
FASCIA LATA

RECTUS FEMORIS

VASTUS LATERALIS
VASTUS INTERMEDIUS

QUADRICEPS

PECTORALIS
MAJOR

SERRATUS
ANTERIOR

LATISSIMUS
DORSI

OBLIQUUS
ABDOMINIS
EXTERNUS

ILIAC CREST

PATELLA

TIBIALIS
ANTERIOR

PERONEUS BREVIS

EXTENSOR
DIGITORUM LONGUS

SOLEUS

PERONEUS LONGUS

GASTROCNEMIUS

SEMIMEMBRANOSUS

SHORT HEAD
BICEPS FEMORIS
LONG HEAD

SEMITENDINOSUS

GLUTEUS MEDIUS

GREATER
TROCHANTER

GLUTEUS MAXIMUS

FASCIA LATA, ILIOTIBIAL TRACT

EXECUTION OF THE MOVEMENT

Begin

End

Sit on the ground leaning on the elbows, knees bent, with the thighs vertical and the lower legs parallel to the floor. Inhale and extend the legs, keeping the feet fairly high off the floor. Return to the initial position with maximum contraction of the abdominal muscles. Exhale at the end of the effort.

This exercise should be performed slowly without jerks. To feel the abdominal muscles working and to avoid lumbar area contractures it is important to gently round the back during the entire execution of this movement. Long series until you feel a burning sensation produce the best results.

This exercise works mainly on the rectus abdominis muscles of the abdomen and to a lesser degree the internal and external obliques of the abdomen as well as the flexor muscle group (tensor fascia lata, rectus femoris, and iliopsoas) and incidentally the pectineus.

9   CRUNCHES ON A WALL BAR

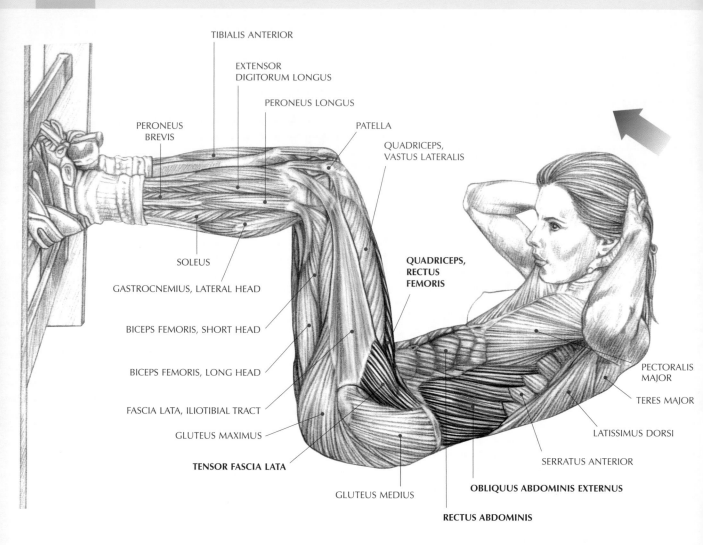

TIBIALIS ANTERIOR

EXTENSOR DIGITORUM LONGUS

PERONEUS LONGUS

PERONEUS BREVIS

PATELLA

QUADRICEPS, VASTUS LATERALIS

SOLEUS

QUADRICEPS, RECTUS FEMORIS

GASTROCNEMIUS, LATERAL HEAD

BICEPS FEMORIS, SHORT HEAD

BICEPS FEMORIS, LONG HEAD

FASCIA LATA, ILIOTIBIAL TRACT

GLUTEUS MAXIMUS

TENSOR FASCIA LATA

GLUTEUS MEDIUS

PECTORALIS MAJOR

TERES MAJOR

LATISSIMUS DORSI

SERRATUS ANTERIOR

OBLIQUUS ABDOMINIS EXTERNUS

RECTUS ABDOMINIS

Wedge the feet in the wall bars, thighs vertical, torso on the ground, hands behind the head. Inhale and raise the torso as high as possible by rounding the back. Exhale at the end of the movement.

This exercise works the rectus abdominis and to a lesser extent the external and internal oblique muscles of the abdomen. Note that by moving the torso farther away from the wall bars and wedging the feet lower, the mobility of the pelvis is increased, allowing for bigger oscillations and better solicitation of the flexor muscles of the hip (iliopsoas, rectus femoris, and tensor fascia lata).

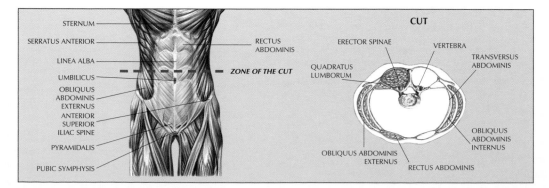

STERNUM

SERRATUS ANTERIOR

LINEA ALBA

UMBILICUS

OBLIQUUS ABDOMINIS EXTERNUS

ANTERIOR SUPERIOR ILIAC SPINE

PYRAMIDALIS

PUBIC SYMPHYSIS

RECTUS ABDOMINIS

ZONE OF THE CUT

CUT

ERECTOR SPINAE

VERTEBRA

QUADRATUS LUMBORUM

TRANSVERSUS ABDOMINIS

OBLIQUUS ABDOMINIS INTERNUS

OBLIQUUS ABDOMINIS EXTERNUS

RECTUS ABDOMINIS

CRUNCHES ON A BENCH

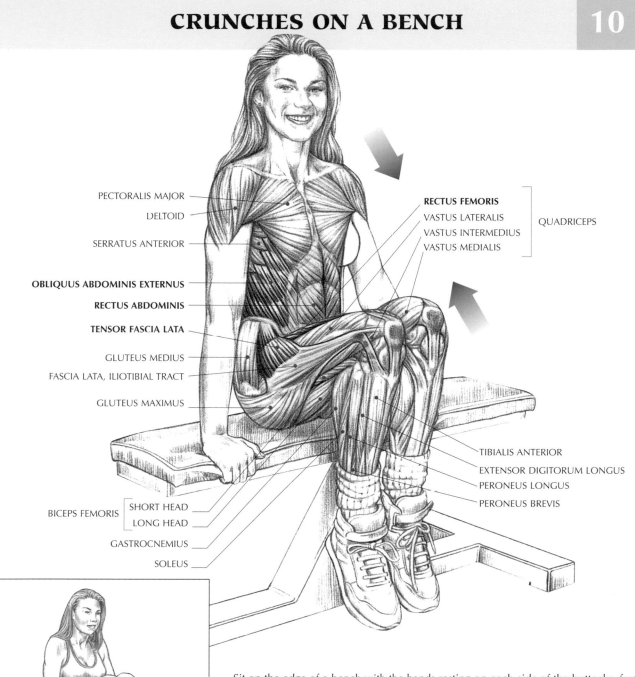

PECTORALIS MAJOR

DELTOID

SERRATUS ANTERIOR

OBLIQUUS ABDOMINIS EXTERNUS

RECTUS ABDOMINIS

TENSOR FASCIA LATA

GLUTEUS MEDIUS

FASCIA LATA, ILIOTIBIAL TRACT

GLUTEUS MAXIMUS

RECTUS FEMORIS

VASTUS LATERALIS

VASTUS INTERMEDIUS

VASTUS MEDIALIS

QUADRICEPS

TIBIALIS ANTERIOR

EXTENSOR DIGITORUM LONGUS

PERONEUS LONGUS

PERONEUS BREVIS

BICEPS FEMORIS
SHORT HEAD
LONG HEAD

GASTROCNEMIUS

SOLEUS

EXECUTION OF THE MOVEMENT

Sit on the edge of a bench with the hands resting on each side of the buttocks, feet off the floor. Inhale and bring the knees to the chest while rounding the back at the same time. Return to the initial position while exhaling, and begin again.

This exercise works mainly the rectus muscles of the abdomen. The external and internal oblique muscles and the flexor muscles of the hip (tensor fascia lata, rectus femoris, and, deeper, the iliopsoas) are also solicited.

Notes
- To feel the rectus muscles of the abdomen working you need to maintain an isometric contraction for one or two seconds at the end of lifting up the knees.
- Series of 20 repetitions give the best results.

11 CRUNCHES ON AN INCLINE BENCH

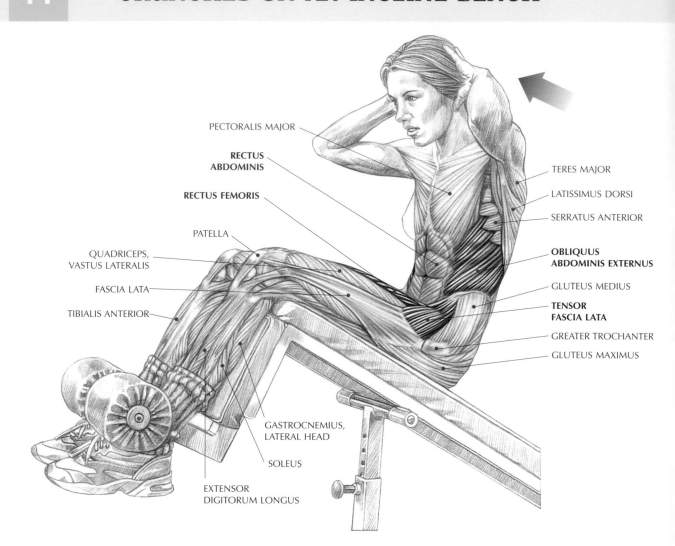

PECTORALIS MAJOR

RECTUS ABDOMINIS

RECTUS FEMORIS

PATELLA

QUADRICEPS, VASTUS LATERALIS

FASCIA LATA

TIBIALIS ANTERIOR

GASTROCNEMIUS, LATERAL HEAD

SOLEUS

EXTENSOR DIGITORUM LONGUS

TERES MAJOR

LATISSIMUS DORSI

SERRATUS ANTERIOR

OBLIQUUS ABDOMINIS EXTERNUS

GLUTEUS MEDIUS

TENSOR FASCIA LATA

GREATER TROCHANTER

GLUTEUS MAXIMUS

Sit on a bench with your feet wedged under the pads, hands behind the head. Inhale and lean back, never more than 20 degrees. Roll back up, rounding the back slightly to target the rectus abdominis better. Exhale at the end of the movement.

This exercise is performed in long series. With it you can work the abdominal group as well as the iliopsoas, the tensor fascia lata, and the rectus femoris; these last three muscles are worked during the forward tilting of the pelvis.

Variation
By rotating the torso while straightening up, part of the effort is placed on the obliques.

Example
Rotation to the left will work the right external oblique and the left internal oblique more intensely, as well as the rectus abdominis on the right side. Torsions are performed either alternately or unilaterally; in any case the goal is to focus on feeling the muscles, and it is of no use to exaggerate the tilt of the back.

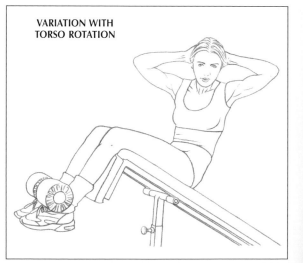

VARIATION WITH TORSO ROTATION

CRUNCHES ON AN INCLINE BOARD

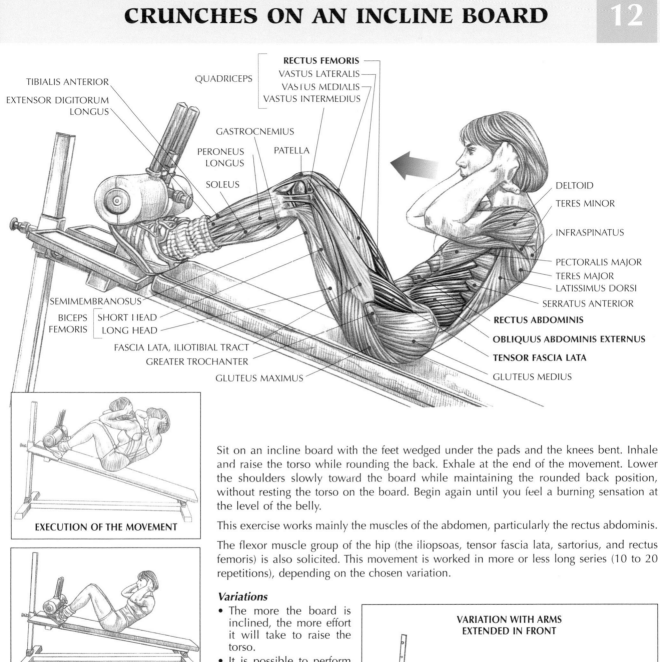

TIBIALIS ANTERIOR
EXTENSOR DIGITORUM LONGUS
QUADRICEPS
RECTUS FEMORIS
VASTUS LATERALIS
VASTUS MEDIALIS
VASTUS INTERMEDIUS
GASTROCNEMIUS
PERONEUS LONGUS
PATELLA
SOLEUS
DELTOID
TERES MINOR
INFRASPINATUS
PECTORALIS MAJOR
TERES MAJOR
LATISSIMUS DORSI
SERRATUS ANTERIOR
RECTUS ABDOMINIS
OBLIQUUS ABDOMINIS EXTERNUS
TENSOR FASCIA LATA
GLUTEUS MEDIUS
SEMIMEMBRANOSUS
BICEPS FEMORIS
SHORT HEAD
LONG HEAD
FASCIA LATA, ILIOTIBIAL TRACT
GREATER TROCHANTER
GLUTEUS MAXIMUS

EXECUTION OF THE MOVEMENT

Sit on an incline board with the feet wedged under the pads and the knees bent. Inhale and raise the torso while rounding the back. Exhale at the end of the movement. Lower the shoulders slowly toward the board while maintaining the rounded back position, without resting the torso on the board. Begin again until you feel a burning sensation at the level of the belly.

This exercise works mainly the muscles of the abdomen, particularly the rectus abdominis.

The flexor muscle group of the hip (the iliopsoas, tensor fascia lata, sartorius, and rectus femoris) is also solicited. This movement is worked in more or less long series (10 to 20 repetitions), depending on the chosen variation.

Variations
- The more the board is inclined, the more effort it will take to raise the torso.
- It is possible to perform the movement in small amplitude (or in small oscillations of the torso) or in greater amplitude by lowering the torso almost to the board.
- For greater ease the exercise may be performed with the arms extended in front.

The more the board is inclined, the more difficult it will be to perform the movement.

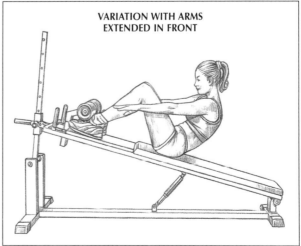

VARIATION WITH ARMS EXTENDED IN FRONT

SUSPENDED CRUNCHES
AT A BENCH

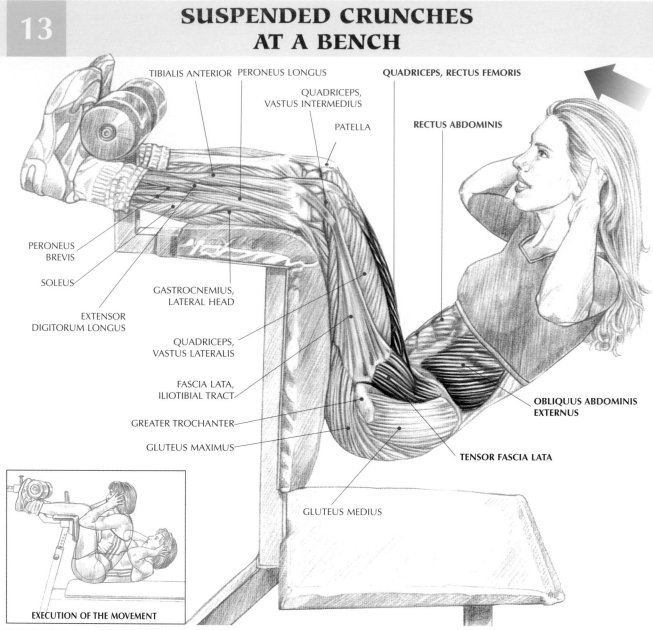

TIBIALIS ANTERIOR

PERONEUS LONGUS

QUADRICEPS, VASTUS INTERMEDIUS

PATELLA

QUADRICEPS, RECTUS FEMORIS

RECTUS ABDOMINIS

PERONEUS BREVIS

SOLEUS

EXTENSOR DIGITORUM LONGUS

GASTROCNEMIUS, LATERAL HEAD

QUADRICEPS, VASTUS LATERALIS

FASCIA LATA, ILIOTIBIAL TRACT

GREATER TROCHANTER

GLUTEUS MAXIMUS

OBLIQUUS ABDOMINIS EXTERNUS

TENSOR FASCIA LATA

GLUTEUS MEDIUS

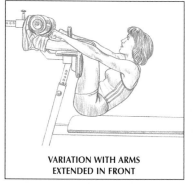

EXECUTION OF THE MOVEMENT

VARIATION WITH ARMS
EXTENDED IN FRONT

Wedge your feet under the pads, with your torso free and your hands behind your head. Inhale and raise your torso, trying to touch your knees with your head, being careful to roll up the spinal column. Exhale at the end of the contraction.

This exercise is excellent for developing the rectus abdominis muscle. It also engages the obliques less intensely. Note that with forward tilting of the pelvis the rectus femoris, iliopsoas, and tensor fascia lata contribute strongly.

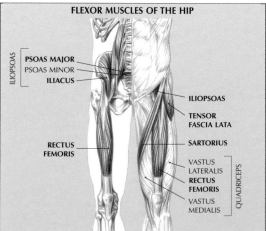

FLEXOR MUSCLES OF THE HIP

ILIOPSOAS

PSOAS MAJOR
PSOAS MINOR
ILIACUS

ILIOPSOAS

TENSOR FASCIA LATA

SARTORIUS

RECTUS FEMORIS

VASTUS LATERALIS
RECTUS FEMORIS
VASTUS MEDIALIS

QUADRICEPS

Note

This movement requires good strength, acquired by first practicing easier exercises.

LEG RAISES
IN AN ABDOMINAL CHAIR

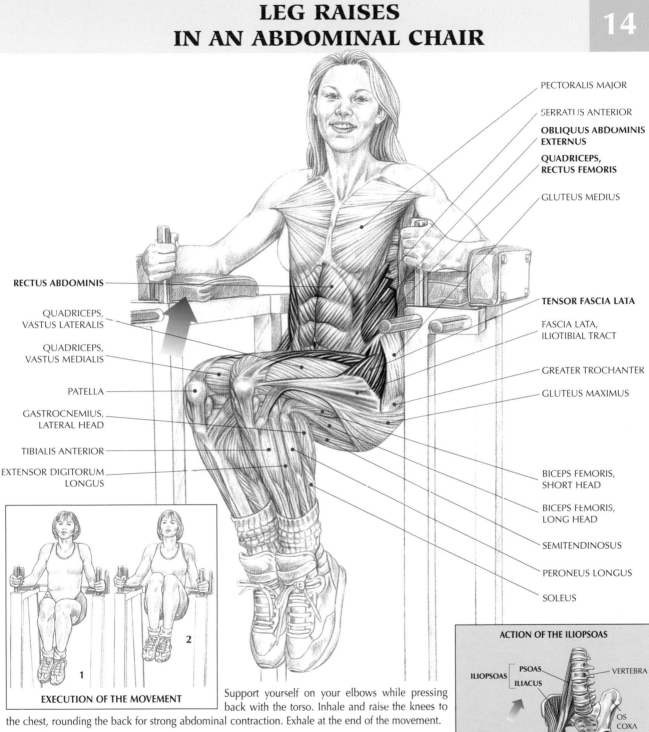

PECTORALIS MAJOR

SERRATUS ANTERIOR

OBLIQUUS ABDOMINIS EXTERNUS

QUADRICEPS, RECTUS FEMORIS

GLUTEUS MEDIUS

RECTUS ABDOMINIS

QUADRICEPS, VASTUS LATERALIS

QUADRICEPS, VASTUS MEDIALIS

PATELLA

GASTROCNEMIUS, LATERAL HEAD

TIBIALIS ANTERIOR

EXTENSOR DIGITORUM LONGUS

TENSOR FASCIA LATA

FASCIA LATA, ILIOTIBIAL TRACT

GREATER TROCHANTER

GLUTEUS MAXIMUS

BICEPS FEMORIS, SHORT HEAD

BICEPS FEMORIS, LONG HEAD

SEMITENDINOSUS

PERONEUS LONGUS

SOLEUS

EXECUTION OF THE MOVEMENT

Support yourself on your elbows while pressing back with the torso. Inhale and raise the knees to the chest, rounding the back for strong abdominal contraction. Exhale at the end of the movement.

This exercise works the flexors of the hip, mainly the iliopsoas, as well as the obliques and rectus abdominis. The latter is intensely solicited in its inferior part.

Variations
- To focus the work on the abdominals, perform small oscillations with the legs, keeping a rounded back and never lowering the knees below horizontal.
- To intensify the effort, perform the movement with the legs extended; this requires good flexibility of the hamstrings.
- Finally you can keep the knees tucked toward the chest with an isometric contraction for a few seconds.

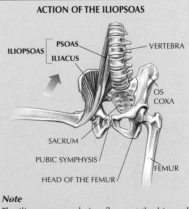

ACTION OF THE ILIOPSOAS

ILIOPSOAS

PSOAS

ILIACUS

VERTEBRA

OS COXA

SACRUM

PUBIC SYMPHYSIS

HEAD OF THE FEMUR

FEMUR

Note
The iliopsoas muscle is a flexor at the hip and an external rotator at the thigh.

15   LEG RAISES FROM A FIXED BAR

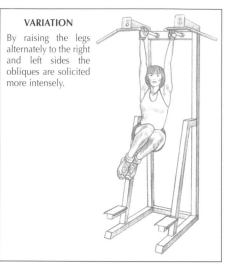

VARIATION
By raising the legs alternately to the right and left sides the obliques are solicited more intensely.

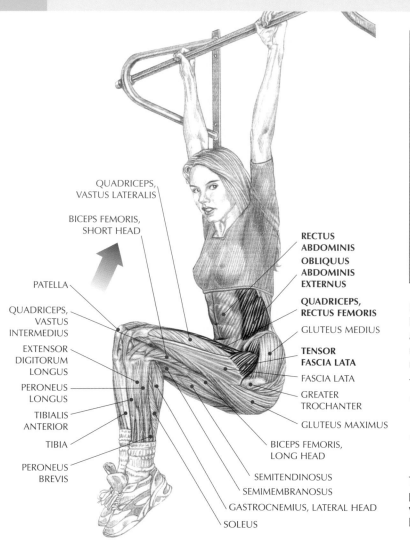

QUADRICEPS, VASTUS LATERALIS

BICEPS FEMORIS, SHORT HEAD

PATELLA

QUADRICEPS, VASTUS INTERMEDIUS

EXTENSOR DIGITORUM LONGUS

PERONEUS LONGUS

TIBIALIS ANTERIOR

TIBIA

PERONEUS BREVIS

RECTUS ABDOMINIS

OBLIQUUS ABDOMINIS EXTERNUS

QUADRICEPS, RECTUS FEMORIS

GLUTEUS MEDIUS

TENSOR FASCIA LATA

FASCIA LATA

GREATER TROCHANTER

GLUTEUS MAXIMUS

BICEPS FEMORIS, LONG HEAD

SEMITENDINOSUS

SEMIMEMBRANOSUS

GASTROCNEMIUS, LATERAL HEAD

SOLEUS

Hang from a fixed bar. Inhale and raise the knees as high as possible, taking care to approximate the pubis to the sternum for a roll-up of the spine. Exhale at the end of the movement.

The action of this exercise targets

- the iliopsoas, the rectus femoris, and the tensor fascia lata when the legs are being raised, and
- the rectus abdominis and to a lesser extent the obliques with the pubis/sternum approximation.

To focus the work on the abdominal muscles, perform small oscillations of the thighs without ever lowering the knees below horizontal.

ABDOMINAL-LUMBAR EQUILIBRIUM

It is important to work the abdominal muscles and the erector spinae in the back in a balanced way. Hypotonicity or hypertonicity of one of these two muscle groups can lead to bad posture, which over time may cause a problem.

Example

Hypertonicity of the lower part of the erector spinae (the lumbosacral mass) associated with hypotonicity of the abdominal muscles will lead to hyperlordosis and abdominal ptosis. This postural fault may, if caught in time, be alleviated with strengthening of the abdominal muscles.

Conversely, hypertonic abdominal muscles associated with relatively slack erector spinae, especially in their upper part (the spinales, longissimus, and iliocostales of the thorax) leads to kyphosis (rounding of the upper back) with loss of the vertebral curves. This postural fault can be alleviated by specific strengthening exercises of the erector spinae.

Hypertonicity of the erector spinae, which leads to hyperlordosis

Hypotonicity of the abdominal muscles leads to ptosis

Rounded kyphosis of the upper back

Hypotonicity of the erector spinae with loss of vertebral curves

Hyper-tonicity of the muscles of the abdomen

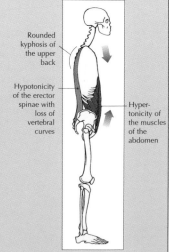

LEG RAISES ON AN INCLINE BOARD
WITH CRUNCHES

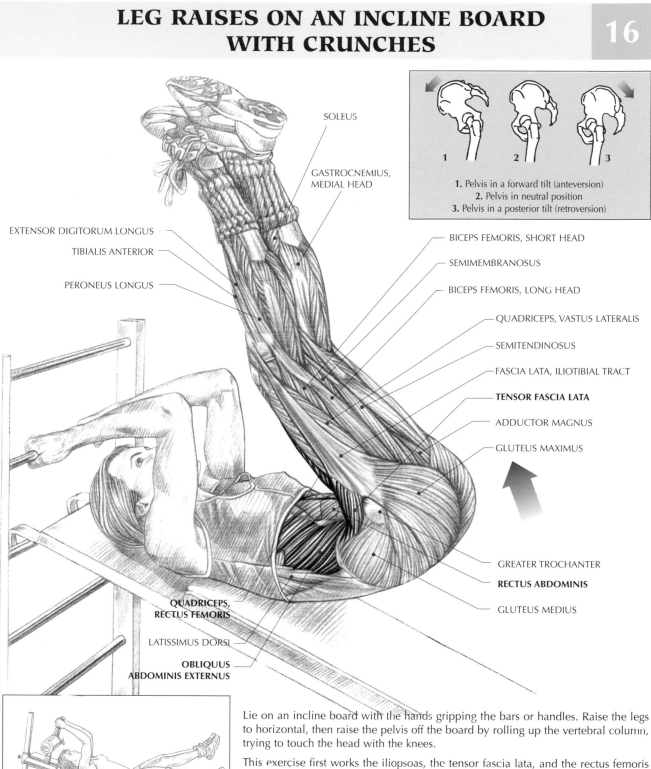

1. Pelvis in a forward tilt (anteversion)
2. Pelvis in neutral position
3. Pelvis in a posterior tilt (retroversion)

SOLEUS

GASTROCNEMIUS, MEDIAL HEAD

EXTENSOR DIGITORUM LONGUS

TIBIALIS ANTERIOR

PERONEUS LONGUS

BICEPS FEMORIS, SHORT HEAD

SEMIMEMBRANOSUS

BICEPS FEMORIS, LONG HEAD

QUADRICEPS, VASTUS LATERALIS

SEMITENDINOSUS

FASCIA LATA, ILIOTIBIAL TRACT

TENSOR FASCIA LATA

ADDUCTOR MAGNUS

GLUTEUS MAXIMUS

GREATER TROCHANTER

RECTUS ABDOMINIS

GLUTEUS MEDIUS

QUADRICEPS, RECTUS FEMORIS

LATISSIMUS DORSI

OBLIQUUS ABDOMINIS EXTERNUS

VARIATION
With smaller oscillations.

Lie on an incline board with the hands gripping the bars or handles. Raise the legs to horizontal, then raise the pelvis off the board by rolling up the vertebral column, trying to touch the head with the knees.

This exercise first works the iliopsoas, the tensor fascia lata, and the rectus femoris of the quadriceps. Secondly, as the hips lift off the board and the spine rolls up, the abdominal muscles are solicited, mainly the rectus abdominis part below the navel.

Note

This is an excellent exercise for people having problems feeling the lower part of the abdominals work. Given the difficulty of the exercise it is recommended that newcomers set the bench at less of an angle.

17 PELVIC LIFTS OFF THE FLOOR

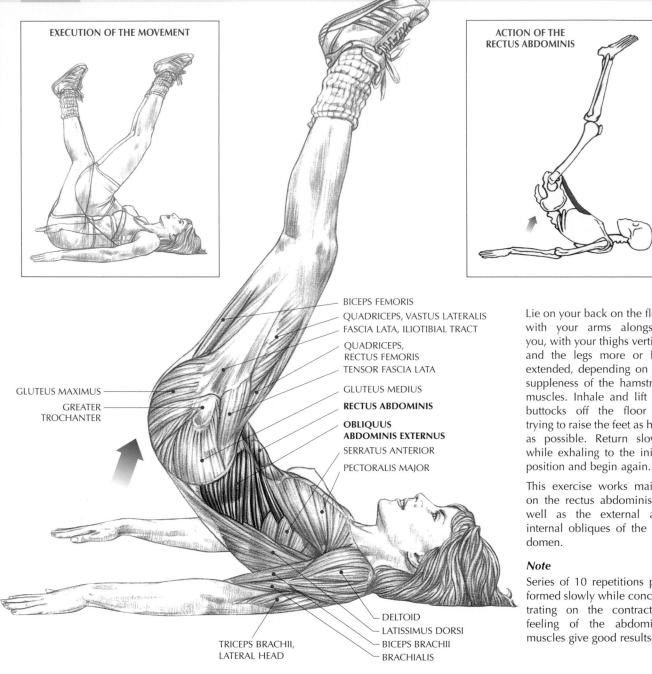

EXECUTION OF THE MOVEMENT

ACTION OF THE RECTUS ABDOMINIS

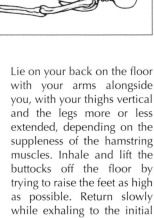

BICEPS FEMORIS
QUADRICEPS, VASTUS LATERALIS
FASCIA LATA, ILIOTIBIAL TRACT
QUADRICEPS, RECTUS FEMORIS
TENSOR FASCIA LATA
GLUTEUS MEDIUS
RECTUS ABDOMINIS
OBLIQUUS ABDOMINIS EXTERNUS
SERRATUS ANTERIOR
PECTORALIS MAJOR

GLUTEUS MAXIMUS
GREATER TROCHANTER

DELTOID
LATISSIMUS DORSI
BICEPS BRACHII
BRACHIALIS

TRICEPS BRACHII, LATERAL HEAD

Lie on your back on the floor with your arms alongside you, with your thighs vertical and the legs more or less extended, depending on the suppleness of the hamstring muscles. Inhale and lift the buttocks off the floor by trying to raise the feet as high as possible. Return slowly while exhaling to the initial position and begin again.

This exercise works mainly on the rectus abdominis as well as the external and internal obliques of the abdomen.

Note
Series of 10 repetitions performed slowly while concentrating on the contraction feeling of the abdominal muscles give good results.

VARIATION WITH LESSER AMPLITUDE

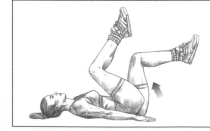

It is possible to perform the movement with lesser amplitude (that is, by raising the pelvis but maintaining the back against the ground). This variation allows the effort to be concentrated on the lower part of the rectus abdominis muscles below the navel.

Series of 20 reps provide the best results.

PELVIC ROTATIONS ON THE FLOOR

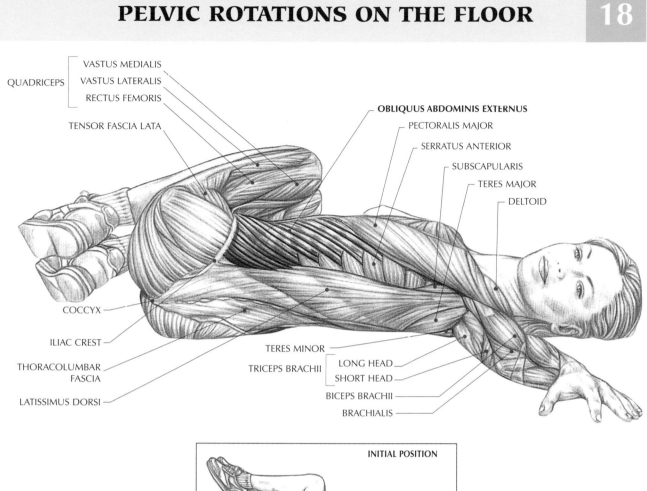

QUADRICEPS
VASTUS MEDIALIS
VASTUS LATERALIS
RECTUS FEMORIS

TENSOR FASCIA LATA

OBLIQUUS ABDOMINIS EXTERNUS

PECTORALIS MAJOR

SERRATUS ANTERIOR

SUBSCAPULARIS

TERES MAJOR

DELTOID

COCCYX

ILIAC CREST

THORACOLUMBAR FASCIA

LATISSIMUS DORSI

TERES MINOR

TRICEPS BRACHII
LONG HEAD
SHORT HEAD

BICEPS BRACHII

BRACHIALIS

INITIAL POSITION

Lie on the floor with your arms extended at shoulder level, thighs vertical, and knees bent. Inhale and slowly lower the legs to the floor while exhaling. Return to the initial position while inhaling, and continue on with the same movement to the other side.

While the hip flexor muscles are engaged in a static contraction, this exercise works mainly on the external and internal oblique muscles of the abdomen as well as the portion of the rectus abdominis muscle below the navel. Long series of 20 to 30 complete rotations performed slowly give the best results.

Note

To perform the movement well and to stretch the oblique muscles properly it is important to maintain the head and shoulders on the floor every time the knees are lowered.

Variations

- For people who are flexible behind their thighs, it is possible to increase the intensity of the work by performing the exercise with extended legs.
- To stretch the oblique muscles a little more, it is suggested to turn the head with each rotation of the pelvis. When the knees rotate to the left, rotate the head to the right. This last variation can be considered a stretch for the obliques and the lumbar region.

19

OBLIQUE CRUNCHES
WITH FEET ON THE FLOOR

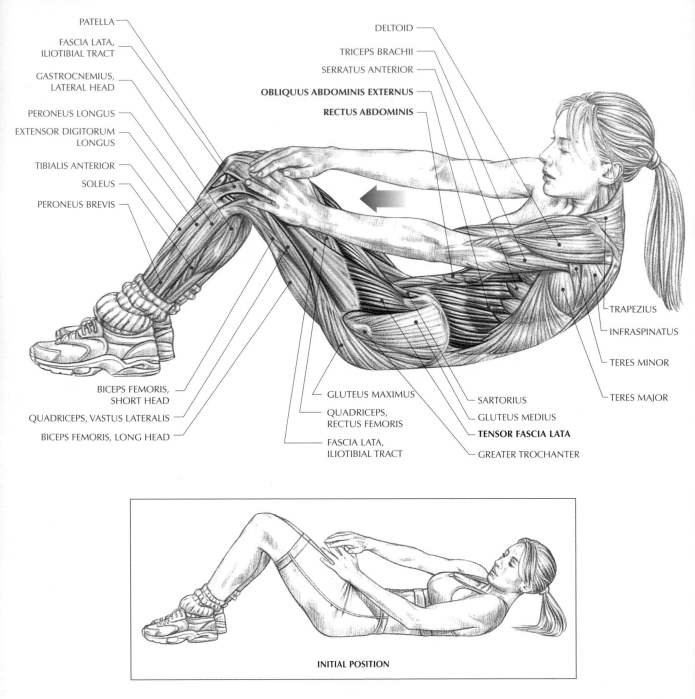

PATELLA

FASCIA LATA,
ILIOTIBIAL TRACT

GASTROCNEMIUS,
LATERAL HEAD

PERONEUS LONGUS

EXTENSOR DIGITORUM
LONGUS

TIBIALIS ANTERIOR

SOLEUS

PERONEUS BREVIS

DELTOID

TRICEPS BRACHII

SERRATUS ANTERIOR

OBLIQUUS ABDOMINIS EXTERNUS

RECTUS ABDOMINIS

TRAPEZIUS

INFRASPINATUS

TERES MINOR

TERES MAJOR

BICEPS FEMORIS,
SHORT HEAD

QUADRICEPS, VASTUS LATERALIS

BICEPS FEMORIS, LONG HEAD

GLUTEUS MAXIMUS

QUADRICEPS,
RECTUS FEMORIS

FASCIA LATA,
ILIOTIBIAL TRACT

SARTORIUS

GLUTEUS MEDIUS

TENSOR FASCIA LATA

GREATER TROCHANTER

INITIAL POSITION

Lie on your back, knees flexed, feet on the floor, arms extended horizontally along one side of your body. Inhale and lift your shoulders off the floor by rounding your back and moving into a slight torsion with your torso to touch the knee with the hands. Exhale at the end of the movement. Return to the initial position but this time rest the torso on the floor. Begin again and alternate from one side to the other until you feel a burn.

This exercise works mainly on the external and internal obliques of the abdomen as well as the rectus abdominis. Because there is weak hip movement the rectus femoris, iliopsoas, and tensor fascia lata are engaged as well but less intensely.

RECOGNIZING THE DIFFERENT KINDS OF ABDOMENS

Flat with little fat is the classic symbol of a toned abdomen. But a certain number of plump people have a toned abdomen, and the only way they will lose their belly is to reduce the thickness of their fat layer by combining a balanced diet with a regular program of physical exercise.

On the other hand a certain number of thin people without excess fat have a protruding belly because of a lack of tone and release of the abdominal muscles. These need to target their training on the abdominal wall with specific exercises aiming at reestablishing postural balance.

SECTION DIAGRAMS OF THE DIFFERENT TYPES OF ABDOMINAL WALLS

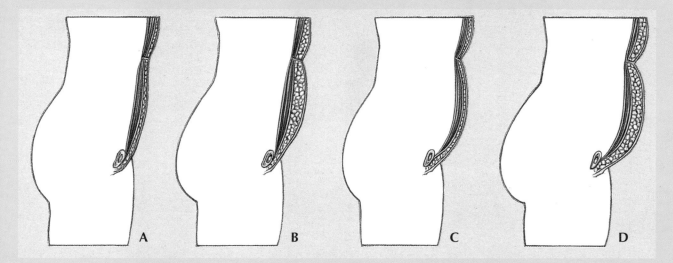

A. Normal abdominal wall with toned muscles.

B. Normal abdominal wall with toned muscles and excess subcutaneous fat giving the impression of ptosis.*

C. Abdominal wall with ptosis because of lack of muscle tone without excess fat.

D. Abdominal wall with ptosis because of lack of muscle tone accompanied by excess fat.

*Ptosis: Inferior displacement of an organ, most often because the structures normally maintaining it have let go. When the abdominal wall lacks tone, it cannot retain the viscera, and the belly collapses and creates a pocket in which the loops of the intestines rest.

20 CYCLING (OR ALTERNATING OBLIQUES) ON THE FLOOR

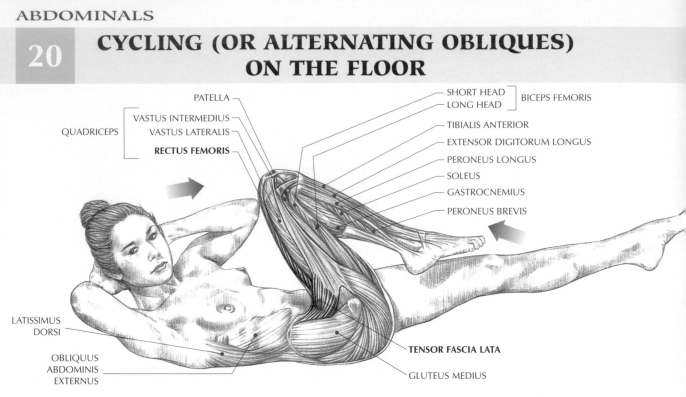

PATELLA

QUADRICEPS
- VASTUS INTERMEDIUS
- VASTUS LATERALIS
- **RECTUS FEMORIS**

SHORT HEAD
LONG HEAD — BICEPS FEMORIS

TIBIALIS ANTERIOR
EXTENSOR DIGITORUM LONGUS
PERONEUS LONGUS
SOLEUS
GASTROCNEMIUS
PERONEUS BREVIS

LATISSIMUS DORSI

OBLIQUUS ABDOMINIS EXTERNUS

TENSOR FASCIA LATA

GLUTEUS MEDIUS

Lie on the floor with your hands behind you at the nape of the neck. Alternate trying to touch opposite knee to elbow from side to side.

To perform the movement well it is important at each elbow-knee touch to roll up the spine by lifting the shoulder off the floor and never to touch the floor with the feet while the legs are in extension. This exercise is executed in long series aiming at a burn sensation at the level of the belly.

The muscles that are mainly engaged are the external and internal obliques and rectus abdominis, and in flexion at the hip the rectus femoris, the tensor fascia lata, the sartorius and, deeper, the iliopsoas muscles.

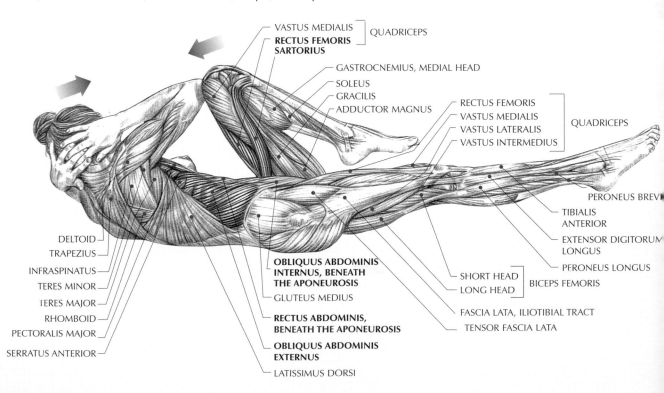

VASTUS MEDIALIS ⎤ QUADRICEPS
**RECTUS FEMORIS
SARTORIUS**

GASTROCNEMIUS, MEDIAL HEAD
SOLEUS
GRACILIS
ADDUCTOR MAGNUS

RECTUS FEMORIS
VASTUS MEDIALIS
VASTUS LATERALIS — QUADRICEPS
VASTUS INTERMEDIUS

PERONEUS BREV
TIBIALIS ANTERIOR
EXTENSOR DIGITORUM LONGUS
PERONEUS LONGUS

SHORT HEAD
LONG HEAD — BICEPS FEMORIS

FASCIA LATA, ILIOTIBIAL TRACT
TENSOR FASCIA LATA

DELTOID
TRAPEZIUS
INFRASPINATUS
TERES MINOR
TERES MAJOR
RHOMBOID
PECTORALIS MAJOR
SERRATUS ANTERIOR

**OBLIQUUS ABDOMINIS
INTERNUS, BENEATH
THE APONEUROSIS**
GLUTEUS MEDIUS

**RECTUS ABDOMINIS,
BENEATH THE APONEUROSIS**

**OBLIQUUS ABDOMINIS
EXTERNUS**

LATISSIMUS DORSI

SIDELYING TORSO FLEXIONS

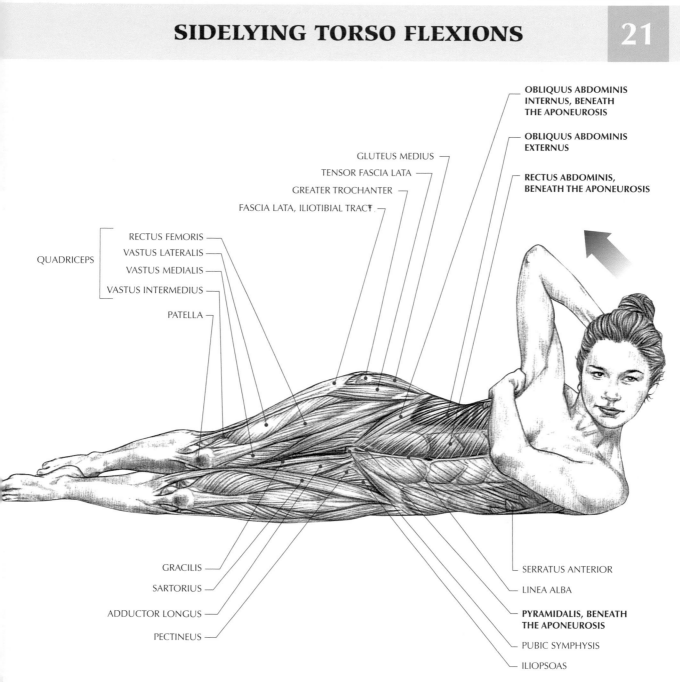

OBLIQUUS ABDOMINIS INTERNUS, BENEATH THE APONEUROSIS

OBLIQUUS ABDOMINIS EXTERNUS

RECTUS ABDOMINIS, BENEATH THE APONEUROSIS

GLUTEUS MEDIUS

TENSOR FASCIA LATA

GREATER TROCHANTER

FASCIA LATA, ILIOTIBIAL TRACT

QUADRICEPS

RECTUS FEMORIS

VASTUS LATERALIS

VASTUS MEDIALIS

VASTUS INTERMEDIUS

PATELLA

GRACILIS

SARTORIUS

ADDUCTOR LONGUS

PECTINEUS

SERRATUS ANTERIOR

LINEA ALBA

PYRAMIDALIS, BENEATH THE APONEUROSIS

PUBIC SYMPHYSIS

ILIOPSOAS

Lie on your side on the floor, legs extended, one hand placed behind the head the other holding onto the side. Perform upward lateral flexion of the torso, trying to lift the shoulder off the floor 10 centimeters. Return to the initial position without resting on the floor and begin again.

This exercise works mainly the external and internal obliques and the rectus abdominis on the flexion side, as well as the quadratus lumborum and to a lesser degree the erector spinae. The movement is performed slowly, always in long series, alternating from side to side until you feel a burn.

Variation
To make it easier it is possible to wedge the feet under furniture or in the gym under wall bars, or to ask a partner to hold the feet.

22 HIGH PULLEY CRUNCHES

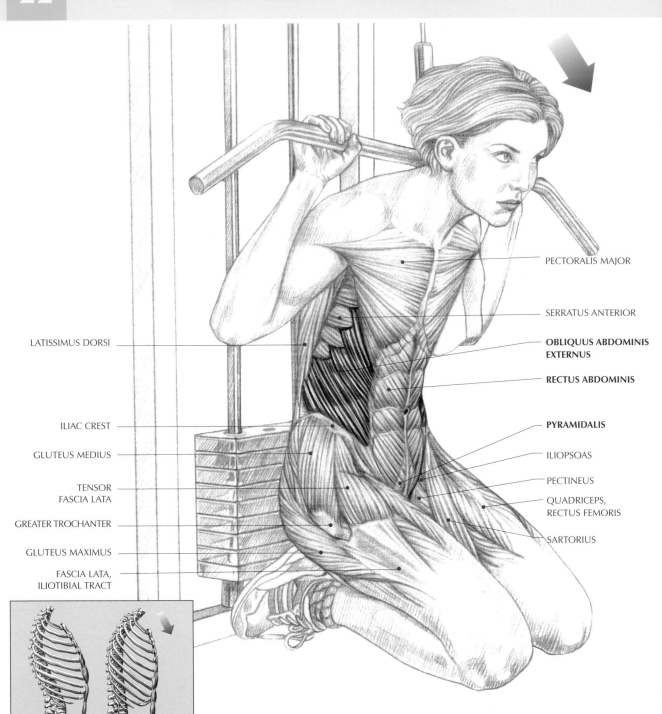

PECTORALIS MAJOR

SERRATUS ANTERIOR

OBLIQUUS ABDOMINIS EXTERNUS

RECTUS ABDOMINIS

PYRAMIDALIS

ILIOPSOAS

PECTINEUS

QUADRICEPS, RECTUS FEMORIS

SARTORIUS

LATISSIMUS DORSI

ILIAC CREST

GLUTEUS MEDIUS

TENSOR FASCIA LATA

GREATER TROCHANTER

GLUTEUS MAXIMUS

FASCIA LATA, ILIOTIBIAL TRACT

ACTION OF THE RECTUS ABDOMINIS

Begin on the knees, with the bar at the nape of the neck. Inhale and round the back to bring the sternum closer to the pubis. Exhale at the end of the movement.

This exercise is never executed with heavy weights; it is important to concentrate on feeling to better focus the work on the abdominal muscles and mainly on the rectus abdominis.

MACHINE CRUNCHES

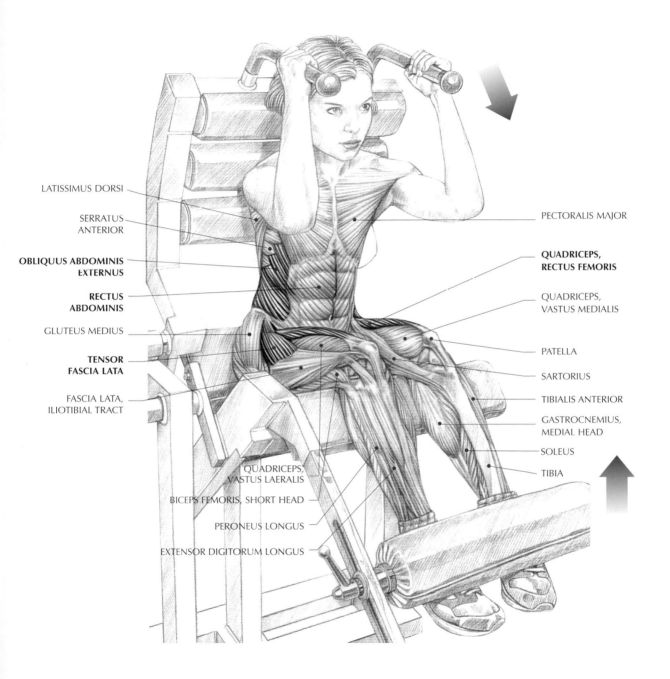

LATISSIMUS DORSI

SERRATUS
ANTERIOR

**OBLIQUUS ABDOMINIS
EXTERNUS**

**RECTUS
ABDOMINIS**

GLUTEUS MEDIUS

**TENSOR
FASCIA LATA**

FASCIA LATA,
ILIOTIBIAL TRACT

QUADRICEPS,
VASTUS LAERALIS

BICEPS FEMORIS, SHORT HEAD

PERONEUS LONGUS

EXTENSOR DIGITORUM LONGUS

PECTORALIS MAJOR

**QUADRICEPS,
RECTUS FEMORIS**

QUADRICEPS,
VASTUS MEDIALIS

PATELLA

SARTORIUS

TIBIALIS ANTERIOR

GASTROCNEMIUS,
MEDIAL HEAD

SOLEUS

TIBIA

Sit at the machine, hands holding the handles, feet wedged under the pads. Inhale and round the spine, trying to approximate the sternum to the pubis as much as possible. Exhale at the end of the movement.

This exercise is excellent as it allows the weights to be adapted to the level of the person. Therefore it can be worked either with light weights for the beginner or with heavy weights without risk for veteran athletes.

24 LATERAL TORSO FLEXIONS ON A BENCH

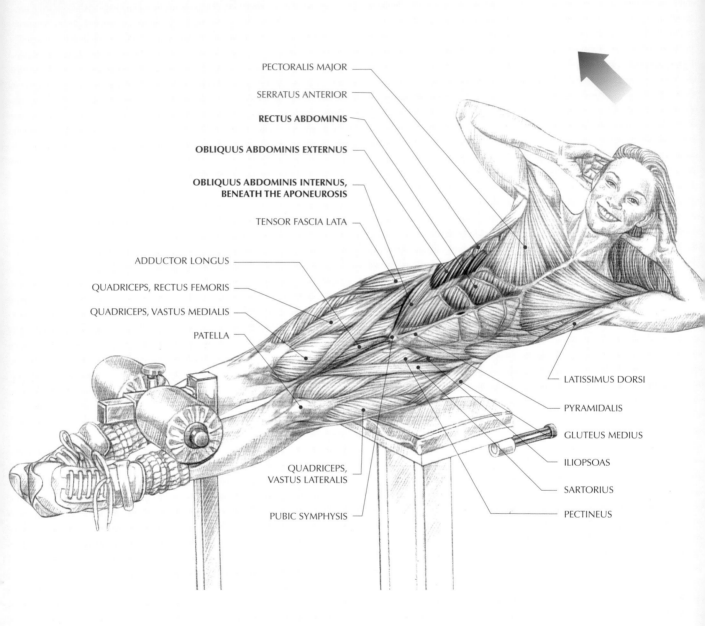

PECTORALIS MAJOR

SERRATUS ANTERIOR

RECTUS ABDOMINIS

OBLIQUUS ABDOMINIS EXTERNUS

OBLIQUUS ABDOMINIS INTERNUS, BENEATH THE APONEUROSIS

TENSOR FASCIA LATA

ADDUCTOR LONGUS

QUADRICEPS, RECTUS FEMORIS

QUADRICEPS, VASTUS MEDIALIS

PATELLA

QUADRICEPS, VASTUS LATERALIS

PUBIC SYMPHYSIS

LATISSIMUS DORSI

PYRAMIDALIS

GLUTEUS MEDIUS

ILIOPSOAS

SARTORIUS

PECTINEUS

This exercise is worked on a bench initially designed for lumbar extensions. Lie on the side, hip on the bench, torso in the air, hands behind the head or on the chest, feet wedged under the pads. Perform lateral flexions of the torso upward.

This movement works mainly on the obliques and the latissimus dorsi on the flexion side, but the obliques and latissimus dorsi on the opposite side are worked in static (isometric) contraction to prevent the torso from dropping below horizontal.

Note
In lateral torso flexions the quadratus lumborum is always solicited.

OBLIQUES AT A ROCKING MACHINE

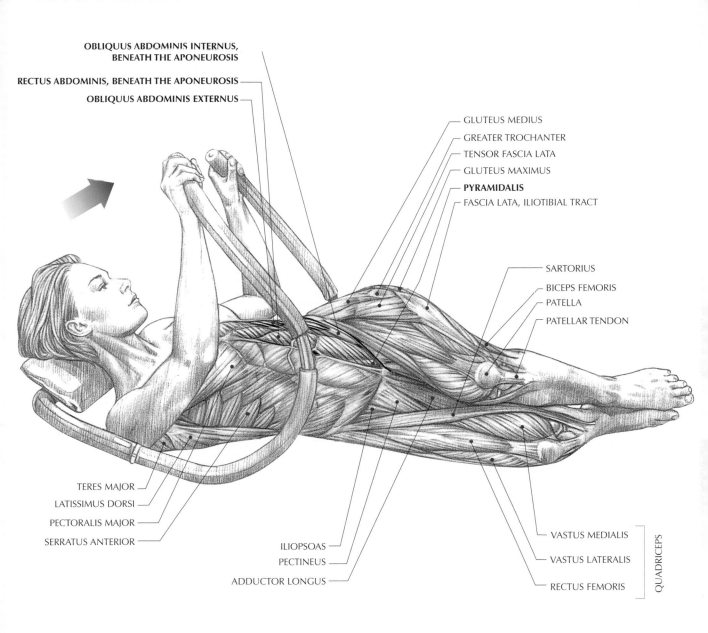

OBLIQUUS ABDOMINIS INTERNUS, BENEATH THE APONEUROSIS

RECTUS ABDOMINIS, BENEATH THE APONEUROSIS

OBLIQUUS ABDOMINIS EXTERNUS

GLUTEUS MEDIUS

GREATER TROCHANTER

TENSOR FASCIA LATA

GLUTEUS MAXIMUS

PYRAMIDALIS

FASCIA LATA, ILIOTIBIAL TRACT

SARTORIUS

BICEPS FEMORIS

PATELLA

PATELLAR TENDON

TERES MAJOR

LATISSIMUS DORSI

PECTORALIS MAJOR

SERRATUS ANTERIOR

ILIOPSOAS

PECTINEUS

ADDUCTOR LONGUS

VASTUS MEDIALIS

VASTUS LATERALIS

RECTUS FEMORIS

QUADRICEPS

Lie on your side, thighs back slightly, knees bent, hands on the upper part of the handles, the head resting on the headrest. Inhale and raise the torso laterally. Exhale at the end of the movement. Return slowly to the initial position and begin again.

This exercise works mainly the internal and external obliques and to a lesser extent the rectus muscles of the abdomen.

26
LATERAL TORSO FLEXIONS
AT A LOW PULLEY

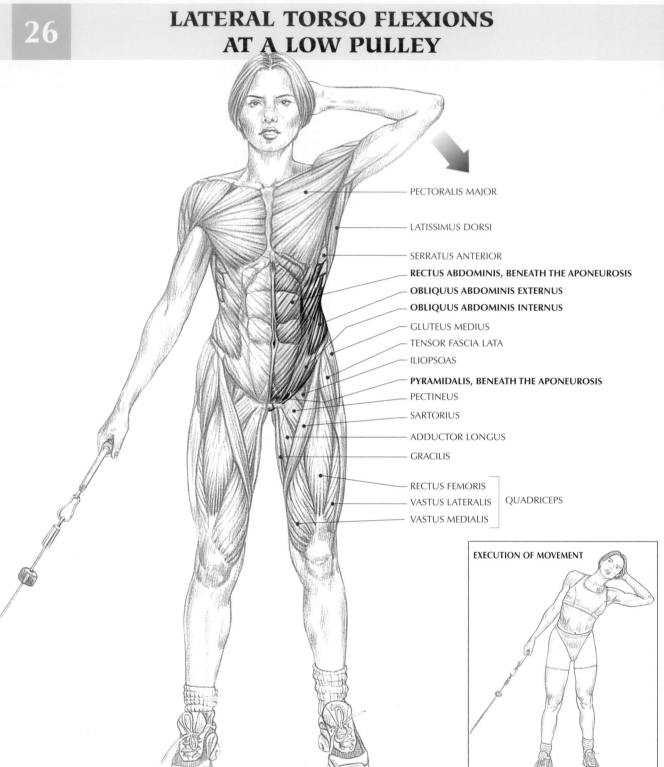

PECTORALIS MAJOR

LATISSIMUS DORSI

SERRATUS ANTERIOR

RECTUS ABDOMINIS, BENEATH THE APONEUROSIS

OBLIQUUS ABDOMINIS EXTERNUS

OBLIQUUS ABDOMINIS INTERNUS

GLUTEUS MEDIUS

TENSOR FASCIA LATA

ILIOPSOAS

PYRAMIDALIS, BENEATH THE APONEUROSIS

PECTINEUS

SARTORIUS

ADDUCTOR LONGUS

GRACILIS

RECTUS FEMORIS

VASTUS LATERALIS — QUADRICEPS

VASTUS MEDIALIS

EXECUTION OF MOVEMENT

Stand with the legs slightly apart, one hand behind the head, grasping the handle of the pulley with the other hand. Perform lateral flexion of the torso to the opposite side of the pulley. Slowly return to the initial position. Alternate series between one side and the other without resting in between.

This movement works mainly on the flexion side on the external and internal oblique muscles of the abdomen, and to a lesser degree the rectus abdominis muscle of the abdomen, the quadratus lumborum muscle, and the deep muscles of the back.

Compared to lateral flexion of the torso with dumbbells, exercising at the pulley makes working with heavier weights easier, which makes it easier to feel the obliques working.

OBLIQUES AT A HIGH PULLEY

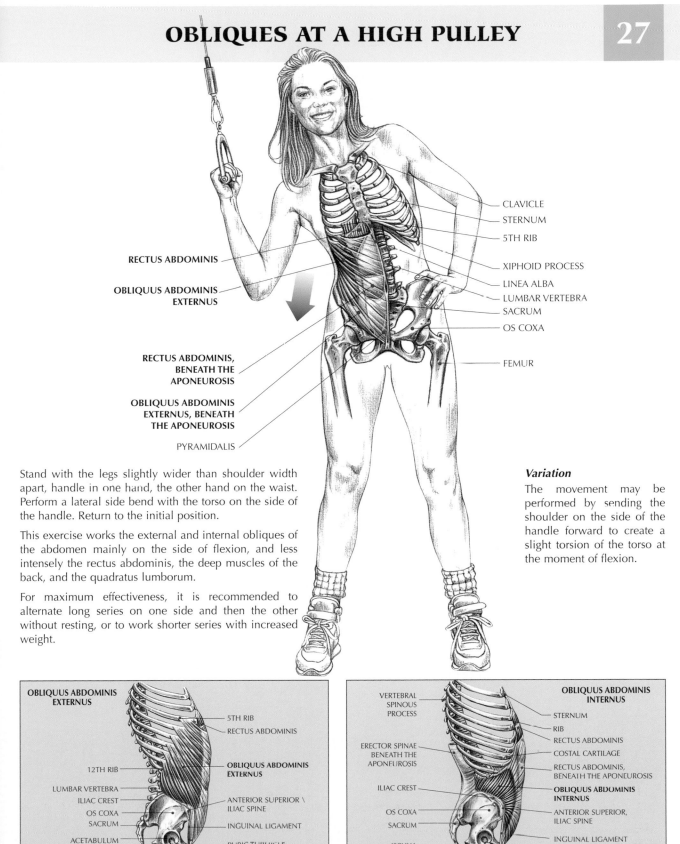

RECTUS ABDOMINIS

OBLIQUUS ABDOMINIS
EXTERNUS

RECTUS ABDOMINIS,
BENEATH THE
APONEUROSIS

OBLIQUUS ABDOMINIS
EXTERNUS, BENEATH
THE APONEUROSIS

PYRAMIDALIS

CLAVICLE
STERNUM
5TH RIB
XIPHOID PROCESS
LINEA ALBA
LUMBAR VERTEBRA
SACRUM
OS COXA
FEMUR

Stand with the legs slightly wider than shoulder width apart, handle in one hand, the other hand on the waist. Perform a lateral side bend with the torso on the side of the handle. Return to the initial position.

This exercise works the external and internal obliques of the abdomen mainly on the side of flexion, and less intensely the rectus abdominis, the deep muscles of the back, and the quadratus lumborum.

For maximum effectiveness, it is recommended to alternate long series on one side and then the other without resting, or to work shorter series with increased weight.

Variation

The movement may be performed by sending the shoulder on the side of the handle forward to create a slight torsion of the torso at the moment of flexion.

OBLIQUUS ABDOMINIS EXTERNUS

5TH RIB
RECTUS ABDOMINIS
OBLIQUUS ABDOMINIS EXTERNUS
12TH RIB
LUMBAR VERTEBRA
ILIAC CREST
OS COXA
SACRUM
ACETABULUM
ANTERIOR SUPERIOR \ ILIAC SPINE
INGUINAL LIGAMENT
PUBIC TUBERCLE

OBLIQUUS ABDOMINIS INTERNUS

VERTEBRAL SPINOUS PROCESS
STERNUM
RIB
RECTUS ABDOMINIS
COSTAL CARTILAGE
ERECTOR SPINAE BENEATH THE APONEUROSIS
RECTUS ABDOMINIS, BENEATH THE APONEUROSIS
OBLIQUUS ABDOMINIS INTERNUS
ILIAC CREST
ANTERIOR SUPERIOR, ILIAC SPINE
OS COXA
SACRUM
ISCHIAL TUBEROSITY
INGUINAL LIGAMENT
PUBIC TUBERCLE

28 LATERAL TORSO FLEXIONS WITH DUMBBELLS

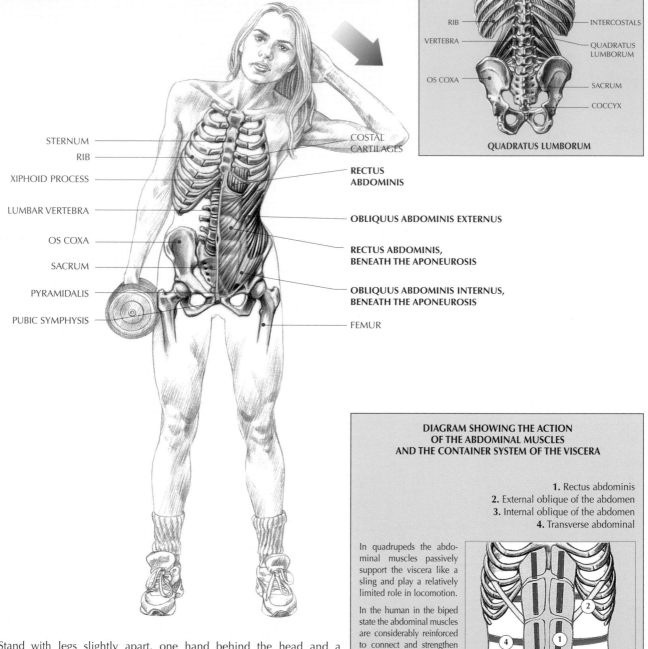

RIB — INTERCOSTALS
VERTEBRA — QUADRATUS LUMBORUM
OS COXA — SACRUM
— COCCYX

QUADRATUS LUMBORUM

STERNUM
RIB
XIPHOID PROCESS
LUMBAR VERTEBRA
OS COXA
SACRUM
PYRAMIDALIS
PUBIC SYMPHYSIS

COSTAL CARTILAGES

RECTUS ABDOMINIS

OBLIQUUS ABDOMINIS EXTERNUS

RECTUS ABDOMINIS, BENEATH THE APONEUROSIS

OBLIQUUS ABDOMINIS INTERNUS, BENEATH THE APONEUROSIS

FEMUR

Stand with legs slightly apart, one hand behind the head and a dumbbell held in the other hand. Perform lateral flexion of the torso to the side opposite the weight. Return to the initial position or beyond, this time with a passive flexion of the torso. Alternate the series, changing the side of the weight without resting.

This exercise mainly works the obliques on the side of flexion, and less intensely the rectus abdominis, the deep muscles of the back, and the quadratus lumborum (the back muscle that inserts onto the twelfth rib and the lumbar transverse processes), as well as the iliac crest.

DIAGRAM SHOWING THE ACTION OF THE ABDOMINAL MUSCLES AND THE CONTAINER SYSTEM OF THE VISCERA

1. Rectus abdominis
2. External oblique of the abdomen
3. Internal oblique of the abdomen
4. Transverse abdominal

In quadrupeds the abdominal muscles passively support the viscera like a sling and play a relatively limited role in locomotion.

In the human in the biped state the abdominal muscles are considerably reinforced to connect and strengthen the pelvis with the torso in the vertical position, to prevent the latter from tilting excessively during walking or running. They have become powerful containing muscles actively wrapping the viscera.

BROOMSTICK TWISTS

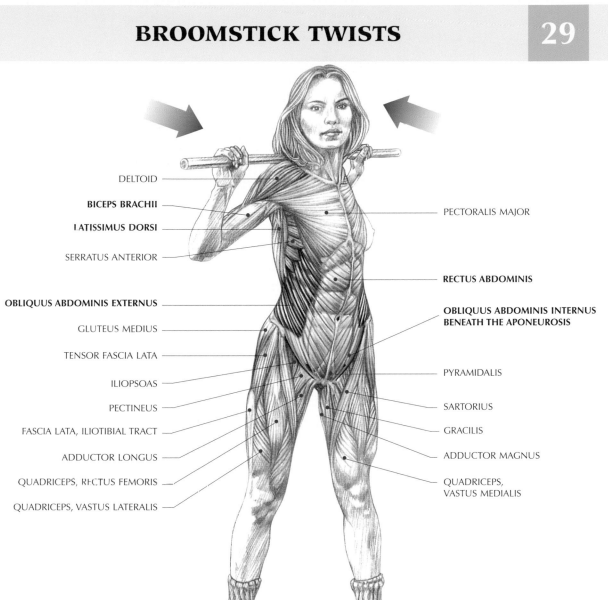

DELTOID

BICEPS BRACHII

LATISSIMUS DORSI

SERRATUS ANTERIOR

OBLIQUUS ABDOMINIS EXTERNUS

GLUTEUS MEDIUS

TENSOR FASCIA LATA

ILIOPSOAS

PECTINEUS

FASCIA LATA, ILIOTIBIAL TRACT

ADDUCTOR LONGUS

QUADRICEPS, RECTUS FEMORIS

QUADRICEPS, VASTUS LATERALIS

PECTORALIS MAJOR

RECTUS ABDOMINIS

OBLIQUUS ABDOMINIS INTERNUS
BENEATH THE APONEUROSIS

PYRAMIDALIS

SARTORIUS

GRACILIS

ADDUCTOR MAGNUS

QUADRICEPS,
VASTUS MEDIALIS

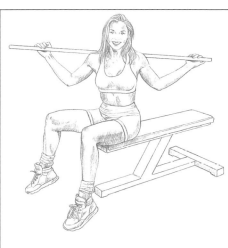

VARIATION SEATED ON A BENCH

Stand with the legs apart, a stick placed at the level of the trapezius above the posterior deltoids, hands resting on the stick without pushing too hard. Perform rotation on the torso from one side to the other, maintaining the pelvis fixed with an isometric contraction of the gluteals.

With the right shoulder forward, this exercise works the right external oblique, the deep left internal oblique, and to a lesser degree the rectus abdominis, the quadratus lumborum, and the extensor muscles of the spine on the left side. For more intensity the back may be slightly rounded. One variation consists of performing the movement seated on a bench, which fixes the pelvis and allows for concentration on the abdominal sling.

Best results are obtained from series of several minutes.

30 SEATED BROOMSTICK TWISTS

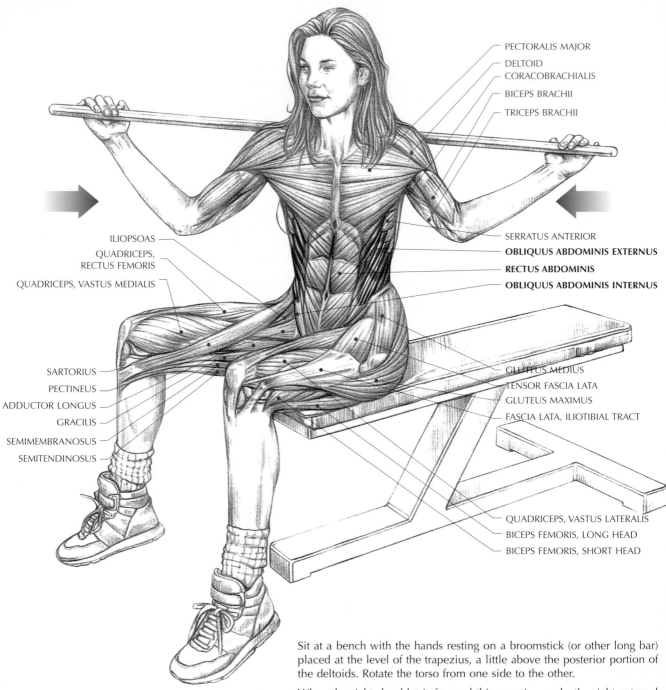

PECTORALIS MAJOR
DELTOID
CORACOBRACHIALIS
BICEPS BRACHII
TRICEPS BRACHII
SERRATUS ANTERIOR
OBLIQUUS ABDOMINIS EXTERNUS
RECTUS ABDOMINIS
OBLIQUUS ABDOMINIS INTERNUS
GLUTEUS MEDIUS
TENSOR FASCIA LATA
GLUTEUS MAXIMUS
FASCIA LATA, ILIOTIBIAL TRACT
QUADRICEPS, VASTUS LATERALIS
BICEPS FEMORIS, LONG HEAD
BICEPS FEMORIS, SHORT HEAD

ILIOPSOAS
QUADRICEPS, RECTUS FEMORIS
QUADRICEPS, VASTUS MEDIALIS
SARTORIUS
PECTINEUS
ADDUCTOR LONGUS
GRACILIS
SEMIMEMBRANOSUS
SEMITENDINOSUS

Sit at a bench with the hands resting on a broomstick (or other long bar) placed at the level of the trapezius, a little above the posterior portion of the deltoids. Rotate the torso from one side to the other.

When the right shoulder is forward this exercise works the right external oblique and, deeper in, the left internal oblique and to a lesser extent the right rectus abdominis, the quadratus lumborum, and the extensor muscles of the spine on the left side. For more intensity, round the back slightly.

Series of several minutes provide the best results. Slow rotations may be alternated with fast rotations during the same series. Example: 100 slow repetitions immediately followed by 50 fast repetitions.

COMPARISON BETWEEN THE TILT OF THE PELVIS IN WOMEN AND MEN

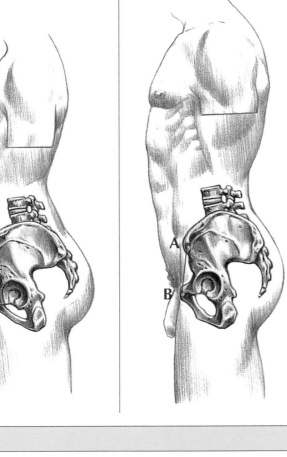

THE TILT OF THE PELVIS

Compared to men, the pelvis in women is generally tilted a little more anteriorly. This anteversion leads to buttocks that are more "pushed out" and a pubis that is more "in" between the thighs, which gives the impression that the lower belly is slightly pushed out. This typical female "pot belly" is in contrast to the vertical abdominal wall more frequent in men, whose pelvis is tilted less forward.

The special position of the pelvis in women during pregnancy helps avoid excessive compression on the viscera by the baby as part of its weight is caught by the abdominal muscles.

A: Anterior superior iliac spine

B: Pubic tubercle

MIDLINE CUT OF THE ABDOMEN OF A PREGNANT WOMAN

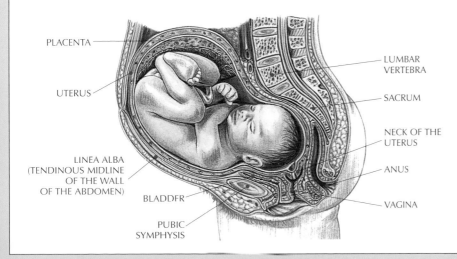

PLACENTA

UTERUS

LINEA ALBA
(TENDINOUS MIDLINE
OF THE WALL
OF THE ABDOMEN)

BLADDER

PUBIC
SYMPHYSIS

LUMBAR
VERTEBRA

SACRUM

NECK OF THE
UTERUS

ANUS

VAGINA

Note
The tilted position of the female pelvis allows part of the weight of the child to be supported by the abdominal muscles. The muscles of the abdominal wall can be compared to a hammock or sling.

31 SEATED TORSO ROTATIONS AT A TWIST MACHINE

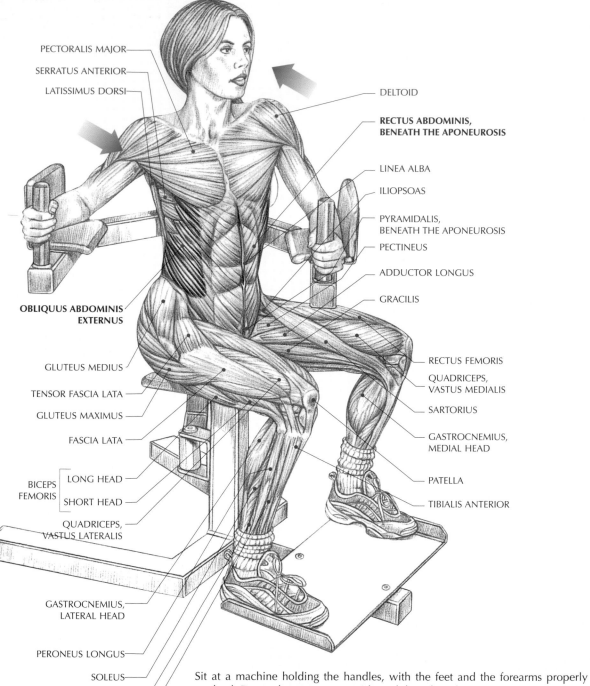

PECTORALIS MAJOR

SERRATUS ANTERIOR

LATISSIMUS DORSI

DELTOID

**RECTUS ABDOMINIS,
BENEATH THE APONEUROSIS**

LINEA ALBA

ILIOPSOAS

PYRAMIDALIS,
BENEATH THE APONEUROSIS

PECTINEUS

ADDUCTOR LONGUS

GRACILIS

**OBLIQUUS ABDOMINIS
EXTERNUS**

RECTUS FEMORIS

QUADRICEPS,
VASTUS MEDIALIS

GLUTEUS MEDIUS

TENSOR FASCIA LATA

SARTORIUS

GLUTEUS MAXIMUS

GASTROCNEMIUS,
MEDIAL HEAD

FASCIA LATA

PATELLA

BICEPS FEMORIS { LONG HEAD

SHORT HEAD

TIBIALIS ANTERIOR

QUADRICEPS,
VASTUS LATERALIS

GASTROCNEMIUS,
LATERAL HEAD

PERONEUS LONGUS

SOLEUS

PERONEUS BREVIS

EXTENSOR DIGITORUM LONGUS

Sit at a machine holding the handles, with the feet and the forearms properly wedged. Rotate the torso to one side and then the other.

When the right shoulder is forward, this exercise works the right external oblique and, deeper, the internal oblique, and to a lesser extent the rectus abdominis, the quadratus lumborum, and the extensors of the spine on the left side.

As with all torso rotations this exercise must be performed without jerking, with a controlled movement. Series for several minutes until a burn is felt provide the best results.

STANDING TORSO ROTATIONS AT A TWIST MACHINE

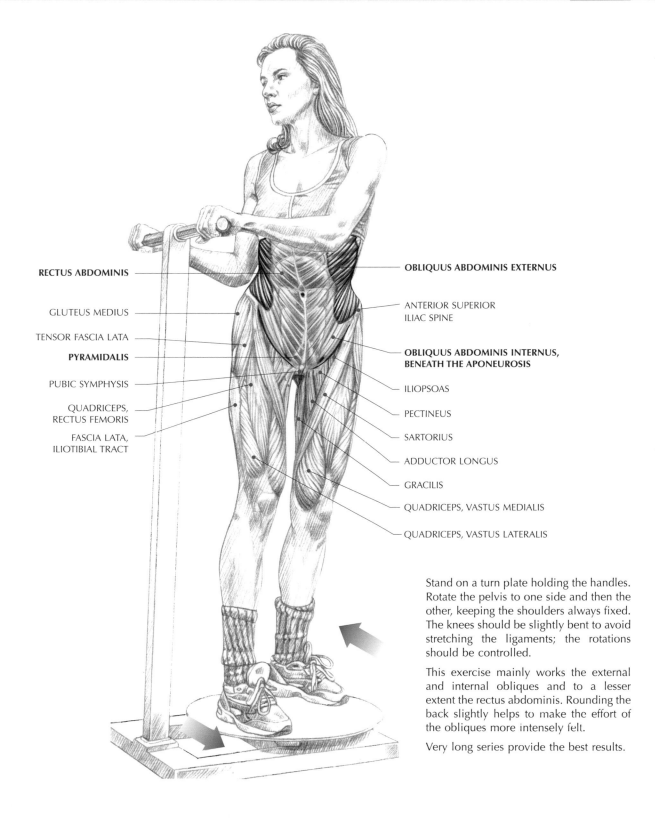

RECTUS ABDOMINIS

GLUTEUS MEDIUS

TENSOR FASCIA LATA

PYRAMIDALIS

PUBIC SYMPHYSIS

QUADRICEPS, RECTUS FEMORIS

FASCIA LATA, ILIOTIBIAL TRACT

OBLIQUUS ABDOMINIS EXTERNUS

ANTERIOR SUPERIOR ILIAC SPINE

OBLIQUUS ABDOMINIS INTERNUS, BENEATH THE APONEUROSIS

ILIOPSOAS

PECTINEUS

SARTORIUS

ADDUCTOR LONGUS

GRACILIS

QUADRICEPS, VASTUS MEDIALIS

QUADRICEPS, VASTUS LATERALIS

Stand on a turn plate holding the handles. Rotate the pelvis to one side and then the other, keeping the shoulders always fixed. The knees should be slightly bent to avoid stretching the ligaments; the rotations should be controlled.

This exercise mainly works the external and internal obliques and to a lesser extent the rectus abdominis. Rounding the back slightly helps to make the effort of the obliques more intensely felt.

Very long series provide the best results.

SEATED TUMMY SUCKS

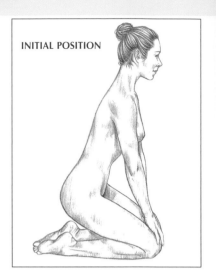

INITIAL POSITION

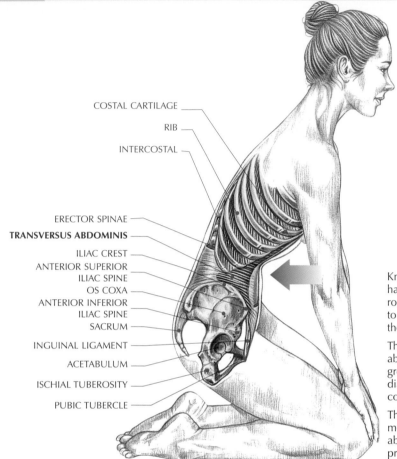

COSTAL CARTILAGE
RIB
INTERCOSTAL

ERECTOR SPINAE
TRANSVERSUS ABDOMINIS
ILIAC CREST
ANTERIOR SUPERIOR ILIAC SPINE
OS COXA
ANTERIOR INFERIOR ILIAC SPINE
SACRUM
INGUINAL LIGAMENT
ACETABULUM
ISCHIAL TUBEROSITY
PUBIC TUBERCLE

Kneel without touching your heels, arms extended, hands leaning on the thighs, the back slightly rounded. Inhale and block the respiration, trying to suck the belly in as much as possible. Return to the initial position while exhaling.

This exercise mainly works the transversus abdominis, which is the deepest of the abdominal group. Its circular and horizontal fibers reduce the diameter of the abdominal region when they contract.

This movement is recommended for young mothers as it helps to tone the transverse abdominal muscles, which are often distended by pregnancy.

Note

Contraction of the transverse muscles of the abdomen is difficult to feel; therefore it is suggested to concentrate on the feeling of the muscle and not on the intensity of the work.

Variation

The transverse muscle can be worked on hands and knees with the back slightly rounded. As in the sitting movement, you need to inhale, block the movement, suck the belly in, and return to the initial position.

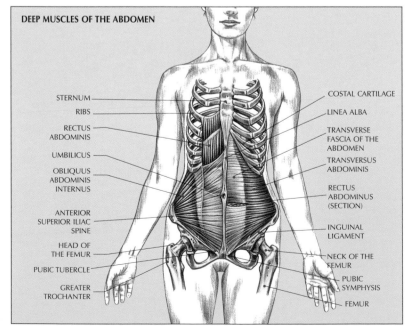

DEEP MUSCLES OF THE ABDOMEN

STERNUM
RIBS
RECTUS ABDOMINIS
UMBILICUS
OBLIQUUS ABDOMINIS INTERNUS
ANTERIOR SUPERIOR ILIAC SPINE
HEAD OF THE FEMUR
PUBIC TUBERCLE
GREATER TROCHANTER

COSTAL CARTILAGE
LINEA ALBA
TRANSVERSE FASCIA OF THE ABDOMEN
TRANSVERSUS ABDOMINIS
RECTUS ABDOMINUS (SECTION)
INGUINAL LIGAMENT
NECK OF THE FEMUR
PUBIC SYMPHYSIS
FEMUR

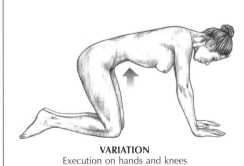

VARIATION
Execution on hands and knees

ABDOMINALS IN HORIZONTAL STABILIZATION

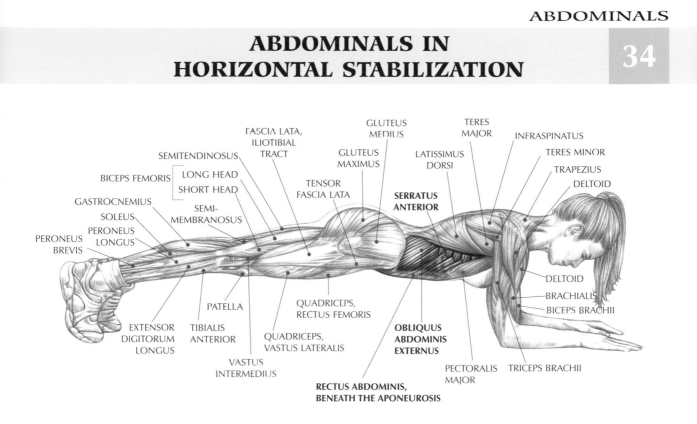

FASCIA LATA, ILIOTIBIAL TRACT

SEMITENDINOSUS

BICEPS FEMORIS

LONG HEAD
SHORT HEAD

GASTROCNEMIUS

SEMI-MEMBRANOSUS

SOLEUS

PERONEUS LONGUS

PERONEUS BREVIS

GLUTEUS MEDIUS

GLUTEUS MAXIMUS

TENSOR FASCIA LATA

TERES MAJOR

LATISSIMUS DORSI

SERRATUS ANTERIOR

INFRASPINATUS

TERES MINOR

TRAPEZIUS

DELTOID

DELTOID

BRACHIALIS

BICEPS BRACHII

EXTENSOR DIGITORUM LONGUS

TIBIALIS ANTERIOR

PATELLA

QUADRICEPS, VASTUS LATERALIS

QUADRICEPS, RECTUS FEMORIS

VASTUS INTERMEDIUS

OBLIQUUS ABDOMINIS EXTERNUS

RECTUS ABDOMINIS, BENEATH THE APONEUROSIS

PECTORALIS MAJOR

TRICEPS BRACHII

Lean on the elbows, palms down, and on the toes, with the body extended as much as possible while trying not to arch the back. Maintain this position for 10 to 30 seconds, breathing normally and facing the floor to avoid excessive tension in the neck.

This "movement" works mainly the rectus muscles of the abdomen as well as the external and internal obliques. While performing this exercise the serratus anterior muscles are also strongly solicited as they maintain the scapulae tight to the rib cage.

Note

Horizontal stabilization is a static, or isometric, exercise (that is to say, the muscle contraction does not produce any articular movement). It is recommended to add it to the training program after having performed the dynamic exercises (that is, articular movements such as the torso raises or crunches).

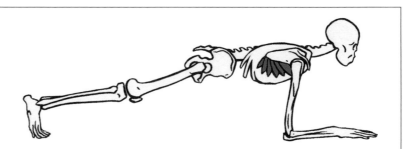

The serratus anterior muscles are strongly engaged to maintain the scapulae tight to the rib cage.

Variations

• To work the oblique muscles of the abdomen more intensely, lateral stabilizations may be performed.

• It is also possible to work dynamically by slowly lowering the pelvis without touching the floor and returning to the initial position. With this variation it is recommended to gently perform series of 10 repetitions.

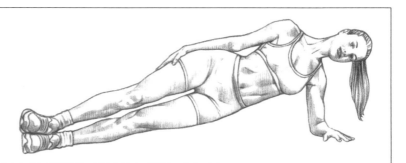

BACK

IV

1. **TORSO EXTENSIONS FROM THE FLOOR**

2. **HORIZONTAL STABILIZATIONS**

3. **TORSO EXTENSIONS ON A BENCH**

4. **DEAD LIFTS**

5. **SUMO-STYLE LIFTS**

6. **TORSO EXTENSIONS AT A MACHINE**

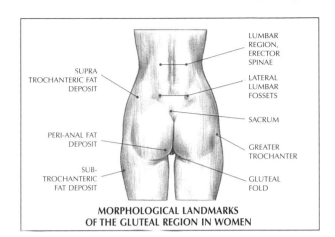

**MORPHOLOGICAL LANDMARKS
OF THE GLUTEAL REGION IN WOMEN**

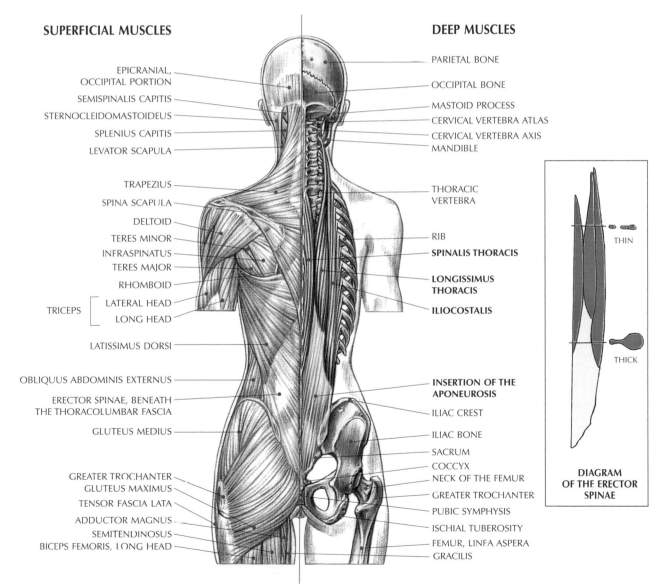

SUPERFICIAL MUSCLES

- EPICRANIAL, OCCIPITAL PORTION
- SEMISPINALIS CAPITIS
- STERNOCLEIDOMASTOIDEUS
- SPLENIUS CAPITIS
- LEVATOR SCAPULA
- TRAPEZIUS
- SPINA SCAPULA
- DELTOID
- TERES MINOR
- INFRASPINATUS
- TERES MAJOR
- RHOMBOID
- TRICEPS
  - LATERAL HEAD
  - LONG HEAD
- LATISSIMUS DORSI
- OBLIQUUS ABDOMINIS EXTERNUS
- ERECTOR SPINAE, BENEATH THE THORACOLUMBAR FASCIA
- GLUTEUS MEDIUS
- GREATER TROCHANTER
- GLUTEUS MAXIMUS
- TENSOR FASCIA LATA
- ADDUCTOR MAGNUS
- SEMITENDINOSUS
- BICEPS FEMORIS, LONG HEAD

DEEP MUSCLES

- PARIETAL BONE
- OCCIPITAL BONE
- MASTOID PROCESS
- CERVICAL VERTEBRA ATLAS
- CERVICAL VERTEBRA AXIS
- MANDIBLE
- THORACIC VERTEBRA
- RIB
- **SPINALIS THORACIS**
- **LONGISSIMUS THORACIS**
- **ILIOCOSTALIS**
- **INSERTION OF THE APONEUROSIS**
- ILIAC CREST
- ILIAC BONE
- SACRUM
- COCCYX
- NECK OF THE FEMUR
- GREATER TROCHANTER
- PUBIC SYMPHYSIS
- ISCHIAL TUBEROSITY
- FEMUR, LINEA ASPERA
- GRACILIS

**DIAGRAM
OF THE ERECTOR
SPINAE**

THIN

THICK

1 TORSO EXTENSIONS FROM THE FLOOR

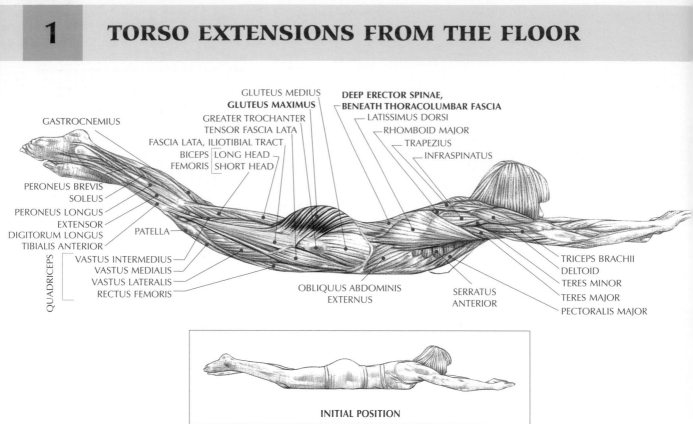

GLUTEUS MEDIUS
GLUTEUS MAXIMUS
GREATER TROCHANTER
TENSOR FASCIA LATA
FASCIA LATA, ILIOTIBIAL TRACT
BICEPS LONG HEAD
FEMORIS SHORT HEAD

**DEEP ERECTOR SPINAE,
BENEATH THORACOLUMBAR FASCIA**
LATISSIMUS DORSI
RHOMBOID MAJOR
TRAPEZIUS
INFRASPINATUS

GASTROCNEMIUS

PERONEUS BREVIS
SOLEUS
PERONEUS LONGUS
EXTENSOR
DIGITORUM LONGUS
TIBIALIS ANTERIOR
PATELLA

QUADRICEPS
VASTUS INTERMEDIUS
VASTUS MEDIALIS
VASTUS LATERALIS
RECTUS FEMORIS

OBLIQUUS ABDOMINIS
EXTERNUS

SERRATUS
ANTERIOR

TRICEPS BRACHII
DELTOID
TERES MINOR
TERES MAJOR
PECTORALIS MAJOR

INITIAL POSITION

Lie prone on the floor with your head raised, looking straight ahead, arms extended slightly off the floor. Extend the torso while simultaneously trying to raise the arms and legs as high as possible. Sustain the contraction a few seconds before returning to the initial position. Slow series of 10 to 15 repetitions give the best results.

This is an excellent exercise without equipment for working the spinal erector muscle group, especially in the lumbar region. The gluteus maximus and the neck (the splenius, the semispinalis, and the clavicular portion of the trapezius) are also worked.

D'ARLOW'S MOVEMENT

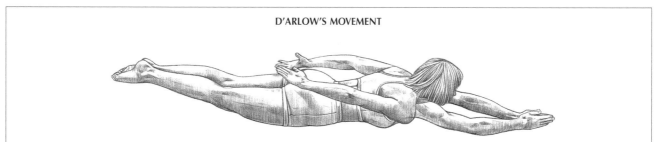

Variation
Lie on your belly on the floor with your head raised and looking straight ahead, back slightly arched, arms and legs extended a few inches off the floor, and hands together. Try to put your hands together behind your back. Return to the initial position without ever touching the floor with either the hands or the feet. Series of 10 to 15 repetitions provide the best results.

As with torso extensions from the floor, this exercise works the spinal erector muscle group, and when the arms approach each other behind the back the rhomboid muscles and the middle and inferior portions of the trapezius are also solicited.

Note
Because of the large range of movement of the arms, people with scapulohumeral pathology (that is, people who suffer from shoulder problems) should not perform this exercise.

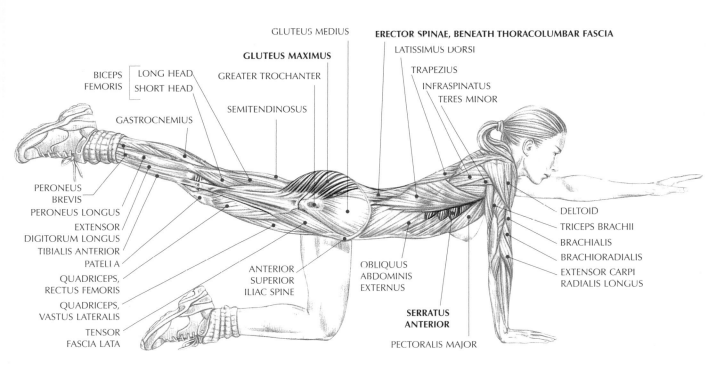

GLUTEUS MEDIUS

ERECTOR SPINAE, BENEATH THORACOLUMBAR FASCIA

LATISSIMUS DORSI

GLUTEUS MAXIMUS

GREATER TROCHANTER

TRAPEZIUS

INFRASPINATUS

TERES MINOR

BICEPS FEMORIS

LONG HEAD

SHORT HEAD

SEMITENDINOSUS

GASTROCNEMIUS

PERONEUS BREVIS

PERONEUS LONGUS

EXTENSOR DIGITORUM LONGUS

TIBIALIS ANTERIOR

PATELLA

QUADRICEPS, RECTUS FEMORIS

QUADRICEPS, VASTUS LATERALIS

TENSOR FASCIA LATA

ANTERIOR SUPERIOR ILIAC SPINE

OBLIQUUS ABDOMINIS EXTERNUS

SERRATUS ANTERIOR

PECTORALIS MAJOR

DELTOID

TRICEPS BRACHII

BRACHIALIS

BRACHIORADIALIS

EXTENSOR CARPI RADIALIS LONGUS

Kneel on the left leg and support yourself on the right hand. Inhale and slowly raise the right leg and left arm, keeping the back as straight as possible. Exhale at the end of the lift.

Maintain this position for 10 to 20 seconds breathing slowly, and then return to the beginning position. Change sides and begin again.

This exercise works the gluteus maximus muscles, the quadratus lumborum, and the erector spinae muscle group (the deep muscles alongside the vertebral column), as well as the deltoids when the arm is raised.

Note that the serratus anterior muscle on the side of the supporting hand is also solicited in order to lock the scapula against the torso.

Variation
This movement may also be practiced by doing alternate raises without stopping at the end of each elevation.

3 TORSO EXTENSIONS ON A BENCH

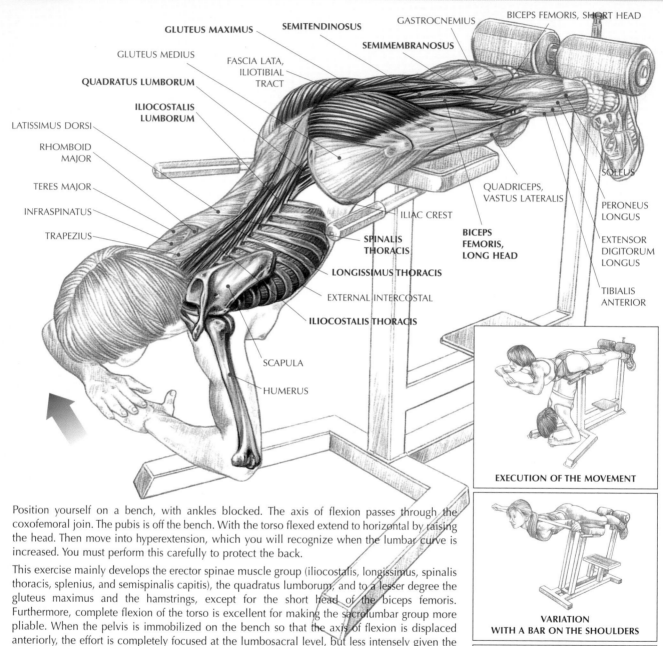

BICEPS FEMORIS, SHORT HEAD
GASTROCNEMIUS
GLUTEUS MAXIMUS
SEMITENDINOSUS
SEMIMEMBRANOSUS
GLUTEUS MEDIUS
FASCIA LATA, ILIOTIBIAL TRACT
QUADRATUS LUMBORUM
ILIOCOSTALIS LUMBORUM
SOLEUS
LATISSIMUS DORSI
RHOMBOID MAJOR
TERES MAJOR
QUADRICEPS, VASTUS LATERALIS
PERONEUS LONGUS
INFRASPINATUS
ILIAC CREST
EXTENSOR DIGITORUM LONGUS
TRAPEZIUS
SPINALIS THORACIS
BICEPS FEMORIS, LONG HEAD
TIBIALIS ANTERIOR
LONGISSIMUS THORACIS
EXTERNAL INTERCOSTAL
ILIOCOSTALIS THORACIS
SCAPULA
HUMERUS

EXECUTION OF THE MOVEMENT

VARIATION WITH A BAR ON THE SHOULDERS

Position yourself on a bench, with ankles blocked. The axis of flexion passes through the coxofemoral join. The pubis is off the bench. With the torso flexed extend to horizontal by raising the head. Then move into hyperextension, which you will recognize when the lumbar curve is increased. You must perform this carefully to protect the back.

This exercise mainly develops the erector spinae muscle group (iliocostalis, longissimus, spinalis thoracis, splenius, and semispinalis capitis), the quadratus lumborum, and to a lesser degree the gluteus maximus and the hamstrings, except for the short head of the biceps femoris. Furthermore, complete flexion of the torso is excellent for making the sacrolumbar group more pliable. When the pelvis is immobilized on the bench so that the axis of flexion is displaced anteriorly, the effort is completely focused at the lumbosacral level, but less intensely given the limited amplitude of movement and the greater force of the lever.

For better focus it is possible at the end of extension to maintain the torso in the horizontal position for a few seconds. An incline bench is recommended for beginners, which makes the performance of this movement more comfortable.

Variations
- When you perform the torso extensions with a bar placed on the shoulders, the upper part is immobilized thereby focusing the effort on the lower part of the erector spinae.
- The specific machine allows the work to be focused on the lumbosacral mass of the spinal muscles.
- For more intensity the movement may be performed with a weight held against the chest or behind the neck.

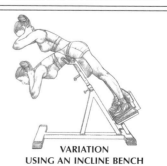

VARIATION USING AN INCLINE BENCH

LOW BACK PAIN

Back pain most commonly affects the lumbar region. Generally speaking, aside from the effects of gravity, low back pain is most often due to cramping of the deep small paravertebral muscles of the back, which mainly connect the osseous processes of the vertebrae.

If during a rotation or an extension of the vertebral column that is poorly controlled the muscle is subjected to excessive stretching or a small tear, it contracts automatically, which at the same time engages the surrounding muscles as well as the more superficial erector muscles. The back is painfully blocked, but at the same time this cramp limits the movements that might tear or aggravate the tear of the muscle.

This contracture, generally of one part of the muscles of the back, lasts some time and most often disappears when the small deep muscle heals. Sometimes, however, the low back pain settles in and, even after healing, local contractures of the back may last for several weeks and, with some people, for years.

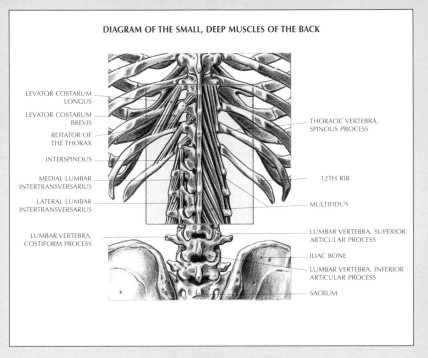

DIAGRAM OF THE SMALL, DEEP MUSCLES OF THE BACK

- LEVATOR COSTARUM LONGUS
- LEVATOR COSTARUM BREVIS
- ROTATOR OF THE THORAX
- INTERSPINOUS
- MEDIAL LUMBAR INTERTRANSVERSARIUS
- LATERAL LUMBAR INTERTRANSVERSARIUS
- LUMBAR VERTEBRA, COSTIFORM PROCESS
- THORACIC VERTEBRA, SPINOUS PROCESS
- 12TH RIB
- MULTIFIDUS
- LUMBAR VERTEBRA, SUPERIOR ARTICULAR PROCESS
- ILIAC BONE
- LUMBAR VERTEBRA, INFERIOR ARTICULAR PROCESS
- SACRUM

Note

When gravity is not the cause, painful contractures of the muscles of the back that characterize low back pain may reflect more serious problems, such as disc herniation, paravertebral muscle, and ligament tears or fractures.

SHOULD YOU ARCH THE BACK?

For those without vertebral pathology, arching the back during an exercise does not carry any risk. On the contrary, with movements such as the squat and the raise off the ground, where the back tends to round, arching the back can prevent injury.

But for certain people, arching the back during an exercise can be very dangerous:

- For people with congenital spondylolysis (absence of fusion of the vertebral arch), extension of the lumbar spine can create a sliding of the vertebra (spondylolysthesis), which can compress the neural elements, leading to sciatica.
- For those who haven't yet finished growing or who are affected with demineralization because of aging (osteoporosis), extension of the lumbar spine can lead to spondylolysis because of fracture of the vertebral arch. When the posterior system for fixing a vertebra has been broken, it can slide and compress the neural elements, leading to sciatica.

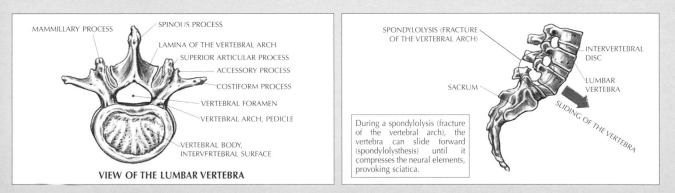

- MAMMILLARY PROCESS
- SPINOUS PROCESS
- LAMINA OF THE VERTEBRAL ARCH
- SUPERIOR ARTICULAR PROCESS
- ACCESSORY PROCESS
- COSTIFORM PROCESS
- VERTEBRAL FORAMEN
- VERTEBRAL ARCH, PEDICLE
- VERTEBRAL BODY, INTERVERTEBRAL SURFACE

VIEW OF THE LUMBAR VERTEBRA

- SPONDYLOLYSIS (FRACTURE OF THE VERTEBRAL ARCH)
- SACRUM
- INTERVERTEBRAL DISC
- LUMBAR VERTEBRA
- SLIDING OF THE VERTEBRA

During a spondylolysis (fracture of the vertebral arch), the vertebra can slide forward (spondylolysthesis) until it compresses the neural elements, provoking sciatica.

4   DEAL LIFTS

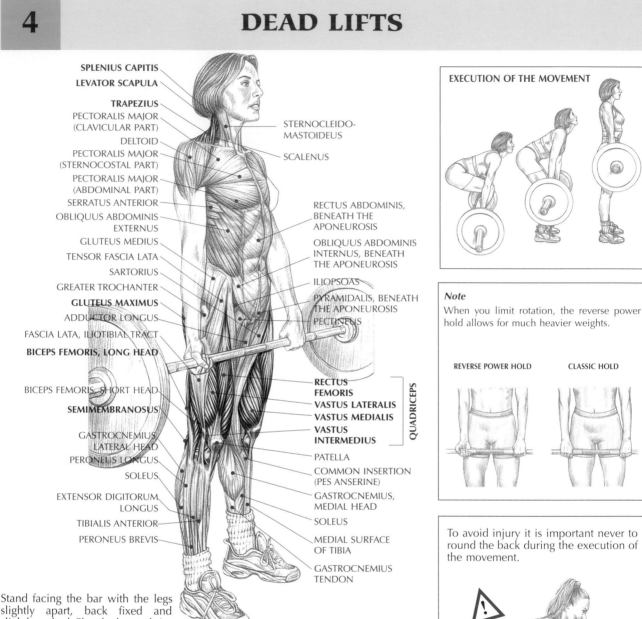

SPLENIUS CAPITIS
LEVATOR SCAPULA
TRAPEZIUS
PECTORALIS MAJOR
(CLAVICULAR PART)
DELTOID
PECTORALIS MAJOR
(STERNOCOSTAL PART)
PECTORALIS MAJOR
(ABDOMINAL PART)
SERRATUS ANTERIOR
OBLIQUUS ABDOMINIS
EXTERNUS
GLUTEUS MEDIUS
TENSOR FASCIA LATA
SARTORIUS
GREATER TROCHANTER
GLUTEUS MAXIMUS
ADDUCTOR LONGUS
FASCIA LATA, ILIOTIBIAL TRACT
BICEPS FEMORIS, LONG HEAD
BICEPS FEMORIS, SHORT HEAD
SEMIMEMBRANOSUS
GASTROCNEMIUS,
LATERAL HEAD
PERONEUS LONGUS
SOLEUS
EXTENSOR DIGITORUM
LONGUS
TIBIALIS ANTERIOR
PERONEUS BREVIS

STERNOCLEIDO-
MASTOIDEUS
SCALENUS
RECTUS ABDOMINIS,
BENEATH THE
APONEUROSIS
OBLIQUUS ABDOMINIS
INTERNUS, BENEATH
THE APONEUROSIS
ILIOPSOAS
PYRAMIDALIS, BENEATH
THE APONEUROSIS
PECTINEUS
RECTUS
FEMORIS
VASTUS LATERALIS
VASTUS MEDIALIS
VASTUS
INTERMEDIUS
}QUADRICEPS
PATELLA
COMMON INSERTION
(PES ANSERINE)
GASTROCNEMIUS,
MEDIAL HEAD
SOLEUS
MEDIAL SURFACE
OF TIBIA
GASTROCNEMIUS
TENDON

EXECUTION OF THE MOVEMENT

Note

When you limit rotation, the reverse power hold allows for much heavier weights.

REVERSE POWER HOLD   CLASSIC HOLD

To avoid injury it is important never to round the back during the execution of the movement.

Stand facing the bar with the legs slightly apart, back fixed and slightly arched. Flex the legs to bring the thighs more or less horizontal; this position is variable depending on the flexibility at the ankles and the morphology of each person (for example, for a person with short femurs and arms, the thighs would be horizontal; for someone with long femurs and arms, the thighs would be a little higher than horizontal). Grasp the bar with the arms extended, hands in an overhand grip a little wider than the shoulders. (By reversing one of the hand holds—one hand in an overhand grip and the other in an underhand grip—you can prevent the bar from rolling, which allows for holding much heavier weights.) Inhale and block the breath, contract the abdominal muscles and the lumbar region, and raise the bar by extending the legs and sliding it along the tibias. When the bar reaches the level of the knees, straighten the torso up completely at the end of extension of the lower extremities; exhale at the end of the effort. Maintain the extension of the body for two seconds and replace the bar, maintaining the abdominal muscle and the lumbar region in contraction.

During the entire execution of the movement it is important never to round the back.

This exercise works all the muscles of the body and has shown to be very effective for developing the lumbosacral and trapezius muscles; the gluteals and quadriceps are also strongly solicited. The lift along with the press and the squat are part of the movements practiced in powerlifting competitions.

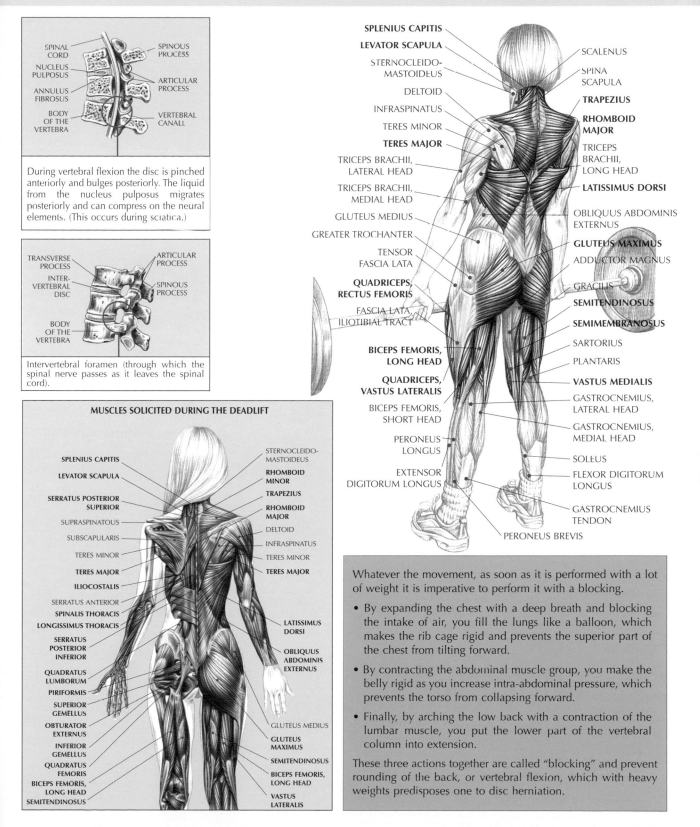

SPINAL CORD · **NUCLEUS PULPOSUS** · **ANNULUS FIBROSUS** · **BODY OF THE VERTEBRA** · **SPINOUS PROCESS** · **ARTICULAR PROCESS** · **VERTEBRAL CANAL**

During vertebral flexion the disc is pinched anteriorly and bulges posteriorly. The liquid from the nucleus pulposus migrates posteriorly and can compress on the neural elements. (This occurs during sciatica.)

TRANSVERSE PROCESS · **INTER-VERTEBRAL DISC** · **BODY OF THE VERTEBRA** · **ARTICULAR PROCESS** · **SPINOUS PROCESS**

Intervertebral foramen (through which the spinal nerve passes as it leaves the spinal cord).

MUSCLES SOLICITED DURING THE DEADLIFT

SPLENIUS CAPITIS · LEVATOR SCAPULA · SERRATUS POSTERIOR SUPERIOR · SUPRASPINATOUS · SUBSCAPULARIS · TERES MINOR · **TERES MAJOR** · **ILIOCOSTALIS** · SERRATUS ANTERIOR · **SPINALIS THORACIS** · **LONGISSIMUS THORACIS** · **SERRATUS POSTERIOR INFERIOR** · **QUADRATUS LUMBORUM** · **PIRIFORMIS** · **SUPERIOR GEMELLUS** · **OBTURATOR EXTERNUS** · **INFERIOR GEMELLUS** · **QUADRATUS FEMORIS** · **BICEPS FEMORIS, LONG HEAD** · **SEMITENDINOSUS**

STERNOCLEIDO-MASTOIDEUS · **RHOMBOID MINOR** · **TRAPEZIUS** · **RHOMBOID MAJOR** · DELTOID · INFRASPINATUS · TERES MINOR · **TERES MAJOR** · **LATISSIMUS DORSI** · **OBLIQUUS ABDOMINIS EXTERNUS** · GLUTEUS MEDIUS · **GLUTEUS MAXIMUS** · **SEMITENDINOSUS** · **BICEPS FEMORIS, LONG HEAD** · **VASTUS LATERALIS**

SPLENIUS CAPITIS · **LEVATOR SCAPULA** · STERNOCLEIDO-MASTOIDEUS · DELTOID · INFRASPINATUS · TERES MINOR · **TERES MAJOR** · TRICEPS BRACHII, LATERAL HEAD · TRICEPS BRACHII, MEDIAL HEAD · GLUTEUS MEDIUS · GREATER TROCHANTER · TENSOR FASCIA LATA · **QUADRICEPS, RECTUS FEMORIS** · FASCIA LATA, ILIOTIBIAL TRACT · **BICEPS FEMORIS, LONG HEAD** · **QUADRICEPS, VASTUS LATERALIS** · BICEPS FEMORIS, SHORT HEAD · PERONEUS LONGUS · EXTENSOR DIGITORUM LONGUS

SCALENUS · SPINA SCAPULA · **TRAPEZIUS** · **RHOMBOID MAJOR** · TRICEPS BRACHII, LONG HEAD · **LATISSIMUS DORSI** · OBLIQUUS ABDOMINIS EXTERNUS · **GLUTEUS MAXIMUS** · ADDUCTOR MAGNUS · GRACILIS · **SEMITENDINOSUS** · **SEMIMEMBRANOSUS** · SARTORIUS · PLANTARIS · **VASTUS MEDIALIS** · GASTROCNEMIUS, LATERAL HEAD · GASTROCNEMIUS, MEDIAL HEAD · SOLEUS · FLEXOR DIGITORUM LONGUS · GASTROCNEMIUS TENDON · PERONEUS BREVIS

Whatever the movement, as soon as it is performed with a lot of weight it is imperative to perform it with a blocking.

- By expanding the chest with a deep breath and blocking the intake of air, you fill the lungs like a balloon, which makes the rib cage rigid and prevents the superior part of the chest from tilting forward.

- By contracting the abdominal muscle group, you make the belly rigid as you increase intra-abdominal pressure, which prevents the torso from collapsing forward.

- Finally, by arching the low back with a contraction of the lumbar muscle, you put the lower part of the vertebral column into extension.

These three actions together are called "blocking" and prevent rounding of the back, or vertebral flexion, which with heavy weights predisposes one to disc herniation.

SUMO-STYLE LIFTS

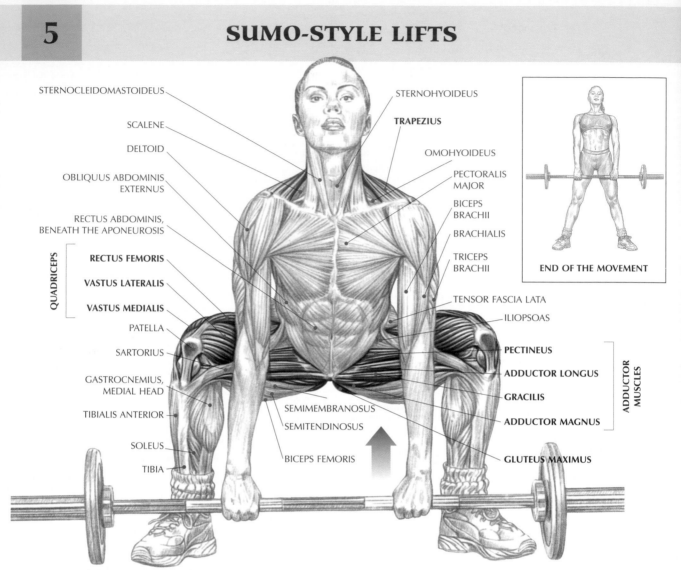

STERNOCLEIDOMASTOIDEUS

SCALENE

DELTOID

OBLIQUUS ABDOMINIS EXTERNUS

RECTUS ABDOMINIS, BENEATH THE APONEUROSIS

QUADRICEPS
RECTUS FEMORIS

VASTUS LATERALIS

VASTUS MEDIALIS

PATELLA

SARTORIUS

GASTROCNEMIUS, MEDIAL HEAD

TIBIALIS ANTERIOR

SOLEUS

TIBIA

STERNOHYOIDEUS

TRAPEZIUS

OMOHYOIDEUS

PECTORALIS MAJOR

BICEPS BRACHII

BRACHIALIS

TRICEPS BRACHII

TENSOR FASCIA LATA

ILIOPSOAS

PECTINEUS

ADDUCTOR LONGUS

GRACILIS

ADDUCTOR MAGNUS

ADDUCTOR MUSCLES

GLUTEUS MAXIMUS

SEMIMEMBRANOSUS

SEMITENDINOSUS

BICEPS FEMORIS

END OF THE MOVEMENT

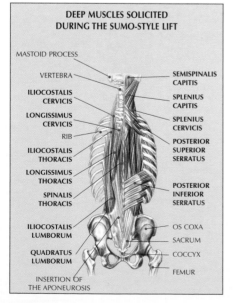

DEEP MUSCLES SOLICITED DURING THE SUMO-STYLE LIFT

MASTOID PROCESS

VERTEBRA

ILIOCOSTALIS CERVICIS

LONGISSIMUS CERVICIS

RIB

ILIOCOSTALIS THORACIS

LONGISSIMUS THORACIS

SPINALIS THORACIS

ILIOCOSTALIS LUMBORUM

QUADRATUS LUMBORUM

INSERTION OF THE APONEUROSIS

SEMISPINALIS CAPITIS

SPLENIUS CAPITIS

SPLENIUS CERVICIS

POSTERIOR SUPERIOR SERRATUS

POSTERIOR INFERIOR SERRATUS

OS COXA

SACRUM

COCCYX

FEMUR

Stand facing the bar, legs slightly spread apart, toes pointed out always in the direction of the knees. Flex the legs to bring the thighs to horizontal; grasp the bar with the arms extended and the hands in an overhand grip more or less shoulder width apart. (By reversing the hold of one hand—one hand either in supination or in an underhand grip and the other in an overhand grip—you prevent the bar from rolling, which allows you to use extremely heavy weights.) Inhale and block the respiration, hollow the back slightly, contract the abdominal muscles, and extend the legs by straightening the torso until you end up in a vertical position with the shoulders pulled back; exhale at the end of the movement. Reposition the bar on the floor, blocking the breathing and never rounding the back.

Unlike the classic lift, this exercise works the quadriceps muscles and the adductor mass of the thighs more intensely and works the back less intensely, as it is less tilted to begin with.

Note

When beginning the movement, it is important to slide the bar along the tibias. When this exercise is practiced in long, light series (maximum 10), it is excellent for strengthening the lumbar region while working the thighs as well as the gluteals.

Nevertheless, with significant weights this movement needs to be performed carefully to avoid damaging the hip joints, the adductor muscles of the thighs, and the lumbosacral hinge, an area that is highly solicited during the execution.

TORSO EXTENSIONS AT A MACHINE

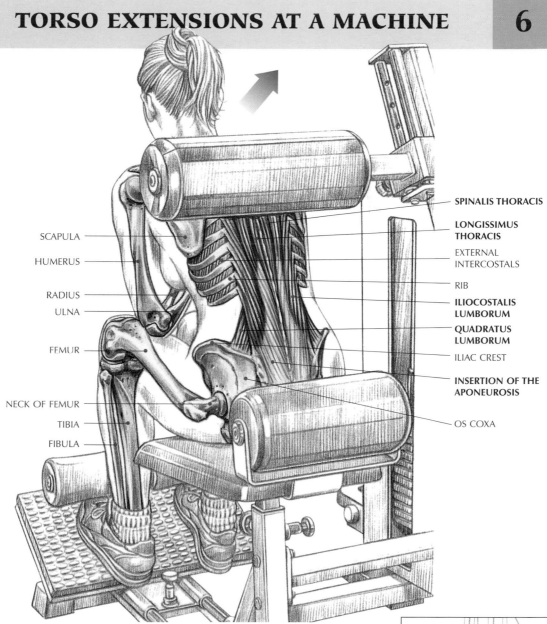

SPINALIS THORACIS

LONGISSIMUS THORACIS

EXTERNAL INTERCOSTALS

RIB

ILIOCOSTALIS LUMBORUM

QUADRATUS LUMBORUM

ILIAC CREST

INSERTION OF THE APONEUROSIS

OS COXA

SCAPULA

HUMERUS

RADIUS

ULNA

FEMUR

NECK OF FEMUR

TIBIA

FIBULA

Sit on the seat of the apparatus, torso tilted forward, the pad of the machine placed at the level of the scapulae. Inhale and straighten the torso as much as possible. Return to the initial position and begin again.

This movement works the erector spinae by concentrating the effort on the lower part of the back (more specifically, on the lumbosacral mass of the spinal muscles).

It is excellent for beginners. It is performed in series of 10 to 20 repetitions and helps develop the strength to move on to more difficult exercises for the back.

This movement can be worked with more weights by reducing the number of repetitions per series. The amplitude of the movement and the weight can be adjusted on the machine; it is possible to change this during the same session.

Example

Two series of 15 repetitions with moderate weights and complete range of performance followed by two series of 7 repetitions with more weights and reduced range.

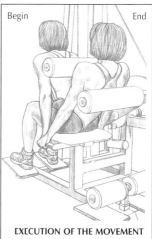

Begin   End

EXECUTION OF THE MOVEMENT

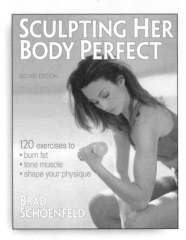
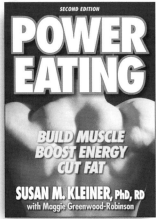
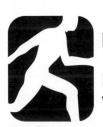